TECHNOLOGY
and the
FUTURE
of Health Care

....

Preparing for the Next 30 Years

David Ellis

with contributions by
Margaret L. Campbell
Donald K. Crandall
Brian E. Peters
Craig Ruff
Kevin L. Seitz
Marianne Udow

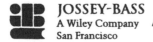

JOSSEY-BASS
A Wiley Company
San Francisco

Health Forum, Inc.
An American Hospital Association Company
CHICAGO press

Jossey-Bass books and products are available through most bookstores. To contact Jossey-Bass directly, call (888) 378-2537, fax to (800) 605-2665, or visit our website at www.josseybass.com.

Substantial discounts on bulk quantities of Jossey-Bass books are available to corporations, professional associations, and other organizations. For details and discount information, contact the special sales department at Jossey-Bass.

This paper is acid-free

TCF and 100 percent totally chlorine-free.

Cover design by Cheri Kusek

Library of Congress Cataloging-in-Publication Data
Ellis, David
  Technology and the future of health care : preparing for the next 30 years / by David Ellis, with contributions by Margaret L. Campbell . . . [et al.].
    p. cm.
  Includes bibliographical references and index.
  ISBN 1-55648-265-5 (hard cover)
  1. Medical technology—Forecasting. 2. Medical innovations—Forecasting. I. Title.
  [DNLM: 1. Technology, Medical. 2. Delivery of Health Care—trends. 3. Forecasting. W 26 E42t 1999]
  R855.3.E44   1999
  610'.28—dc21
  DNLM/DLC
  for Library of Congress   99-40553
                                                                  CIP

HB Printing   10 9 8 7 6 5 4 3 2

CONTENTS

ABOUT THE AUTHORS

David Ellis, technology trends writer, consultant, and public speaker, the founder and former president of Voyager Information Networks, holds a master's degree in the information and communication sciences from Ball State University. Before founding Voyager in 1989, he lived and worked extensively in Europe (Germany and his native England), the Far East (Malaysia, Singapore, and Hong Kong), and the United States (Hawaii, Indiana, and Michigan). His eclectic career path in intelligence, scholarly publishing, strategic consulting, and business leadership reflects a lifelong interest in their common core: information and communication.

Mr. Ellis has written papers and delivered presentations on the future of computing and telecommunications for numerous organizations and in 1998 was invited to address a meeting of the World Technology Network at the Royal Society in London on the topic of the impact of artificial intelligence on business. He is currently writing a book about the past, present, and future of intelligent machines as well as a fictional novel borrowing from his ideas about that future.

Margaret L. Campbell, RN, has been the palliative care nurse practitioner at Detroit Receiving Hospital since 1988. From 1974 to 1988 she served in a number of critical care nursing positions, including staff nurse, educator, and clinical nurse specialist. She is a faculty member at the Wayne State University College of Nursing and School of Medicine. She is a past president of the Medical Ethics Resource Network of Michigan and a member of the Advisory Board to the American Nurses Association Center for Ethics and Human Rights. She served on the Institute of Medicine Committee on Care at the End of Life, which produced the book *Approaching Death: Improving Care at the End of Life.* Ms. Campbell is widely published on care of the dying patient in the acute care setting and is the author of the book *Foregoing Life-Sustaining Therapy: How to Care for the Patient Who Is Near Death,* published by the American Association of Critical-Care Nurses in 1998.

Donald K. Crandall, MD, FACS, is vice president, clinical informatics, at Mercy Health Services in Farmington Hills, Michigan. He graduated from the University of Michigan Medical School in 1963, practiced surgery with Muskegon Surgical Associates in Michigan from 1970 to 1998, and, after graduating from an Advance Training Program in Health Quality Improvement at Intermountain Health in Salt Lake City, became director of the Center for Healthcare Improvement at Mercy General Health Partners in Muskegon before accepting his present appointment.

He has served on various local, state, and national boards, including the Michigan State Medical Society (president, 1983) and the American Medical Association House of Delegates (member, 1977–1992, with service on the Council of Medical Service, dealing with issues related to the practice of medicine). He was also a member of the steering committee of the Health Policy Agenda for the American People, which developed long-range policy direction for the health care industry, and has chaired the Integrated Information Systems Leadership Team of the Muskegon Community Health Project, charged with development of a community-wide health information system.

Brian E. Peters, MHSA, director of corporate initiatives, Michigan Health & Hospital Association (MHA), serves as the association's staff to the Council of Physicians, the Council on Small or Rural Hospitals, and the Council on Osteopathic Health Care. In addition, he assists in the development of the MHA Environmental Assessment and delivers presentations on the future of health care to various audiences. He worked extensively on MHA's *Health Care 2000* and *Next Wave* visioning projects, including studies of the Canadian and British health care systems. He is a member of the Davenport College (Lansing) Physical Therapy Assistant Advisory Board and has served as the treasurer of the Michigan Rural Health Association and the coordinator of the Michigan Organization of Nurse Executives. Mr. Peters holds a master's degree in health services administration from the University of Michigan and a bachelor's degree in business administration from Michigan State University. He completed the Health Executive's Development Program at Cornell University.

Craig Ruff is CEO and president of Public Sector Consultants, Inc., in Lansing, Michigan. Prior to joining the firm, he spent 11 years in the state of Michigan's executive office as special assistant to Gov. William G. Milliken for human services and chief of staff to Lt. Gov. James H. Brickley. He developed legislation, coordinated interdepartmental policies, reviewed agency budgets, and worked closely with numerous professional associations and interest groups. Mr. Ruff has been president of Public Sector Consultants since 1986. As senior consultant to many of the firm's clients, he directs research studies, develops promotional and advocacy strategies, and oversees the management of specific issues for clients. He has authored research studies and publications on health care and public policy issues. He attended the University of Michigan, earning a B.A. in political science and a master's degree in public policy studies.

Kevin L. Seitz is vice president of PPO and ancillary services, Blue Cross and Blue Shield of Michigan. Before joining the Blues in March 1991, Kevin Seitz was director of the Medicaid program for the state of Michigan. Prior to that, he was associate director of human services in the Fiscal Agency of the Michigan House of Representatives. He served as planning and research associate for the Michigan League for Human Services and was a caseworker for the New York City Health and Hospital Corporation. He received a master's degree in social work from the University of Michigan and a bachelor's degree in economics from Hobart College. He serves on the board of directors of the Michigan League for Human Services and the Michigan Council for Maternal and Child Health. He has received the Friends of Nursing Award from the Michigan Nurses Association and was named one of the 500 most influential policymakers in the United States by the editors of *Medicine and Health* magazine.

Marianne Udow is senior vice president of health care products and provider services, Blue Cross and Blue Shield of Michigan. Prior to her present appointment, she was senior vice president of corporate strategy and health care administration and, prior to that, senior vice president of planning and development services. She has also been senior vice president of the Planning and Operations Division at Mercy Alternative Health Systems. She has a master's degree in health services from the University of Michigan School of Public Health. Ms. Udow is board

••

chair of Michigan's Children, an independent, citizen-based child advocacy organization, and is a board member of the Michigan Women's Foundation and a cochair of its Women's Health Funding Initiative committee. She also serves on the Health Care Advisory Board of Enterprise Development Fund. She is a vice president and corporate board member of the Greater Detroit Area Health Council and member of the board of trustees of the Institute for Health Improvement in Southeast Michigan. She has published and been recognized nationally for her contributions to health and women's issues.

ABOUT THE REFERENCES AND NOTES

Much of the research for this book was conducted on the Internet. Documents on the Internet are sometimes deleted, replaced, or moved to another site. Sites themselves can come and go. Where a URL (Internet address) is cited in the endnotes to each chapter, it was valid as of sometime between February 1998 and February 1999, but there is no guarantee it will remain valid. If you seek to link to a URL that returns a "Document not available" message, by typing identifying keywords into one or more of the major search engines (AltaVista, Lycos, InfoSeek, Yahoo, Excite, and so on) you may still be able to locate the document or site. In some cases, I have retained electronic copies of documents and will entertain e-mail requests for assistance in locating source material cited in the endnotes to my chapters. I would also welcome reader comments by e-mail. I can be reached at david@mikiko.net.

ACKNOWLEDGMENTS

I am indebted to the following friends and colleagues for reviewing and commenting on various drafts of this work and for mentoring, motivating, and supporting me through this and various other writing, speaking, and business endeavors. All have contributed to making it a better book, but none shares blame for its inadequacies.

Pamela Shaheen, DrPH, Michigan Public Health Institute. It was Pam's suggestion, encouragement, and practical support that led to the paper from which sprang this book. I am grateful to Pam also for introducing and helping persuade several of the contributing authors to write chapters.

Paul Shaheen, Michigan Council for Maternal and Child Health; Patricia Grauer, MA, Michigan State University College of Osteopathic Medicine; B. Ray Horn, PhD.

My spouse Mikiko has been a loving and immeasurably helpful support throughout.

Richard Hill, editorial director at AHA Press, bore the trials and tribulations of editorship with fortitude, grace, and courtesy. I am grateful to him for recognizing the importance of the topic and encouraging the book's publication.

To Meg Campbell, Don Crandall, Brian Peters, Craig Ruff, Kevin Seitz, and Marianne Udow go my gratitude for their contributions and my admiration at the vision, courage, and leadership expressed through their readiness to participate in what has the potential to turn into a contentious and controversial, but necessary, debate about the future of their professions.

P resenting what may read like science fiction to an audience of clinical minds is a daunting and perilous task, but that is what this book sets out to do. It seeks to show the reader that by taking the known acceleration in technology development of the past 30 years and applying it to the next 30, what reads like science fiction has a reasonable chance of becoming science fact. Make no mistake; I am talking about androids and cyborgs.

I am emboldened in this risky endeavor by the words of futurist consultant and author Peter Schwartz: "The single most frequent failure in the history of forecasting has been grossly underestimating the impact of technologies."[1]

In the past 30 years computers have increasingly and significantly changed our society, and over the past five years the Internet has further accelerated the change. No segment of society and no field of human endeavor has been left untouched by advances in computers and computer-related technologies. The medical profession has experienced many of these changes and is one of the leading adopters of, and innovators in, technology.

To the outside observer, perhaps the most visible changes in medicine are those wrought by such high-tech hardware as MRI, CAT, and PET scanners, but there is a great deal more to it than that. Technology has streamlined the administration of the hospital and the doctor's office, enabling more efficient and cost-effective processing and storage of patient medical and billing records. Telemedicine has advanced to the point where remote specialist consultation can take place through videoconferencing and the immediate transmission of x-ray and other images. Technology has brought noninvasive diagnostic and surgical tools to the physician's practice. And breakthroughs in medicine through computer-assisted research have reduced the half-life of medical knowledge to five or fewer years (my guess); but if there is one thing for sure, it is that technological change will continue to affect the field of medicine and will continue to accelerate.

But more often than not the physician and the nurse, like most of the rest of society, are accelerating at a slower pace and learn of advanced technologies only after the fact of their deployment, leaving them with the problem of adapting quickly to new techniques and leaving the administrator with the problem of altering plans and budgets in order to acquire and install the newly available technology.

To adapt more readily, everyone needs a sense of technological perspective, a "big picture" context within which to plan and conduct his or her career, practice, and continuing education. That perspective can be supplied through an explanation of technology trends and a discussion of their implications. The context is of concern to the medical and nursing practitioner, researcher, and student, as well as to administrators and funding agencies as they formulate policy and make strategic plans for the allocation of resources.

Predicting trends in technology is not an exact science. As John Naisbitt noted in *Megatrends*, attempting to describe the future in detail is the stuff of science fiction, not science.[2] However, through the type of content analysis pioneered by Naisbitt and the scientific discipline known as "futures studies," it is possible to infer and perhaps even to influence broad future trends. These methods involve the synthesis of historical data with empirically derived projections and sometimes with expert anecdotal projections to derive one or more future scenarios.

"The fact that telecommuting has got off to a slow start doesn't mean it is not happening," rightly says economics writer Diane Coyle.[3] But she spoils it by adding: "It is just that organizational change occurs very much more slowly than technological change," claiming that it takes 40 years for an organization to change. I cannot agree with this time estimate, coming as it does at the end of a five-year period covering the infancy of the World Wide Web—a period that has seen a large retail chain, Egghead Software, shut all of its stores and transfer all of its business online. It is, however, self-evident that organizations do usually take longer to change than individuals. Coyle again is correct in noting that "Economic revolutions bring incredible dislocations. Industries vanish and new ones emerge. People are more likely to have to do different work, work in different ways or places. The skills they need for their own prosperity will change."[4]

The key point is that *accelerating* technological change forces *accelerating* organizational (and individual) change, but there is a lag between the two, and when the lag grows big enough, something has to give: either change must decelerate or the organization (and the individual) must accelerate faster. I do not accept the claim that revolutionary change is inherently unpredictable. A substantial increase over the next four decades in the average age of the population could surely be considered a revolutionary change, yet it "can be predicted *with near certainty*," Coyle herself emphasizes.[5]

The fact is, every human-inspired revolution *must* have been predicted, otherwise it could not have occurred. The medium is the message. The difficulty is in getting people to listen.

True revolutions bring change if not progress. People may dispute the very notion of progress, but nobody doubts that things do change over time, even without revolution. This book is concerned with how much and how fast things will change over the next 30 years in the field of health care as a result of accelerating technological trends. The central edifice of health care being (for the moment) the practice of medicine, it is the physician, the patient, and the relationship between them that will bear the brunt of change.

But the same technology trends that have an impact on the physician, the patient, and their relationship also, to a greater or lesser extent, influence the nurse, hospital auxiliary, receptionist, insurer's actuary, civil servant in the government health department, hospital board trustee, health policymaker, and everyone else involved in maintaining a health care system that is a complex of relationships among all of them.

Some of these changes will impact the individual directly; others will be affected through their organizations. The hospital, the clinic, the insurance company, the health professionals' organization, and the government department of health cannot escape the changes, though being thicker-skinned than the individual they may be slower to perceive the impact, and being thicker-skulled they may be slower to react. Perception and reaction are enhanced through expectation. Forewarned is forearmed for the individual as well as the organization. But for forewarning to have practical value, it has to point to action one can take now. The crux of the matter is to differentiate between need-to-know and nice-to-know information.

This is a policy-oriented book about the long term. That is its focus, and therein lies its unique value relative to most health care technology books. Books such as *The Systems Challenge*[6] are practice-oriented books focused on the immediate future. They are "instrumental" books that seek to change immediate practice or behavior. They are good and necessary books, but for leaders concerned about survival in the longer term, they are not sufficient.

This is a "conceptual" book intended to change thinking, which may also lead to changes in practice but in a slower, more subtle, yet ultimately more important way.

The instrumental *versus* conceptual typology of information has long been applied in the social sciences to differentiate between the types of information sought and used by managers on the one hand and by leaders on the other. To use a military analogy, the captain needs instrumental information to carry out his or her primarily tactical mission, whereas the general needs conceptual information for strategy formulation.

This is not to imply that captains don't read conceptual books. The clever and ambitious ones do. But the generals have little taste for instrumental detail and tend not to want too much specificity. This is more than just opinion; it is supported by the voluminous research literature in the field of "knowledge utilization," of which my master's thesis forms a part.

Leaders are keenly interested in what other leaders think, which is one reason the book includes contributions from some nationally recognized leaders in health care. Given the demands on their time, their readiness to contribute to writing the book is the clearest possible evidence of their readiness to read such a book.

The critical need-to-know aspects of this book boil down to two: the *rate of change* and the *impact of change*.

Everybody knows that change is fast and accelerating, but for critical investment and planning decisions to be made, health care leaders need to know how fast and at what rate of acceleration. It is as though we are at the wheel of an automobile without brakes or speedometer and with the gas pedal moving towards the floor of its own volition. We are vaguely alarmed that the highway infrastructure ahead of us may not be able to handle our increasing speed, though we have the means to plan for a safe future infrastructure today—if only we knew what our current speed is and at what rate we are accelerating.

The recent AHA Press book *Change Drivers* set out "to outline the parameters by which the next generation of technologically empowered providers can move ahead and stay ahead in a rapidly expanding marketplace."[7] Indeed, I think it handles the issue of next-generation information systems with aplomb, but since it does not take full and rigorous account of the rate of change (relying, like everyone else, on such generalizations as "existing information systems are being dismantled and reengineered at breakneck speed" and "changes in management practices [are] sweeping through the U.S. economy"), its message is perishable over the longer term.

Nevertheless, in his introduction Roy Ziegler clearly recognizes and succinctly states the problem: "[M]anagers and executives . . . will have to become accustomed to, and learn to shape and direct, the constant change fostered by the rapid evolution of information technology."[8] This book, I hope, will help them to anticipate change by providing an exemplary (not exhaustive) study of computer-based, health care–related technologies.

The first part of this book, "Trends in Technology," illustrates the rate of change in technology over the past 30 years and explains why health professionals need to be cognizant of these changes. It indulges in specific forecasting for technologies that impact change and arrives thereby at an unsettling but nevertheless possible scenario of a radically different medical world in 30 years' time.

Chapter 1 examines the rate of change in general and charts the exponential rate of change in computer and network technologies in particular, since it is these two technologies that underpin and drive trends in the development of all other technologies. Eight key trends are identified and discussed in chapter 2, with examples to illustrate how the trends are surfacing in health care applications. In chapter 3, we begin to focus more specifically on trends in technology-driven health care applications, starting with the technologies of health care administration and control: personal and organizational assistants based on automatic speech and handwriting recognition, natural language processing, machine translation, intelligent agents, smart cards and databases, and smart buildings.

Chapter 4 makes the point that faults, failures, and false starts in these technologies *do not matter* in the context of the next 30 years of accelerated technological development because the research to fix the faults and improve on the technologies is itself accelerating, largely through complexity-busting artificial intelligence–based methods—expert systems, neural nets, and evolutionary systems, which are described and discussed along with some other state-of-the-art technologies useful to health care research; in particular, virtual reality, haptics, and *in silico* experimentation.

Health care delivery products and services emerging from the accelerated R&D discussed in chapter 4 are described in chapter 5. They range from "smart" intensive care units and operating rooms to non-invasive surgeries, surgical nanomachines, biomolecular and genetic therapies, brain implants, and telemedicine. By the time we reach chapter 6, we have all the pieces needed to assemble the inevitable and unavoidable topic of discussion: androids and cyborgs—humanoid robots and robotic people.

Part 1 closes with a discussion, in chapter 7, of some of the more obvious implications of the accelerating pace of technologically driven developments in health care. Because it is a goal of the book to go beyond conceptualizing to advocate instrumental action in the form of an exhaustive and ongoing health care futures study and debate, part 2, "Professional Perspectives," gets the debate rolling. Several nationally known leaders in the health care field were invited to comment on an early draft paper that subsequently formed the basis for this book. Their comments comprise the chapters of part 2.

There is, it seems to me, both enough agreement on some aspects of my thesis and enough disagreement on others that continuance of the debate would be worthwhile. We all seem to agree, for example, that there is a distinct trend toward patient self-management or what some call *consumerism,* and the implications of this alone are worthy of deeper scrutiny by the entire health care community. Some of my contributors disagree with me about the rapidity and/or the strength of the impact that I predict will result from technological acceleration; also reason enough to continue this debate, because getting the answer right is important to all our futures.

Dr. Donald Crandall, a distinguished surgeon, opens the debate (I confess I was relieved to find) by substantially sharing my prognosis for the future of health care in chapter 8, "The Process of the Health Care Encounter." For those seeking "instrumental" action, Don has some excellent suggestions.

Meg Campbell, appropriately for one who has had an exemplary career in nursing, gets up close and personal in that encounter in chapter 9, "Impact of Technology on Nursing Care."

Brian Peters, who leads the Health Care Futures division of the Michigan Health & Hospital Association, steps back to take a broader view in chapter 10, "Hospitals and the Forces of Change."

Blue Cross and Blue Shield of Michigan's Marianne Udow and Kevin Seitz question some of the assumptions and hype surrounding technology developments in chapter 11, "A Payer's Perspective on the Future."

In chapter 12, "Leadership, Followership, and Science," Craig Ruff, CEO of Michigan's leading public policy think tank, stresses the unprecedented power to influence the future that is now available to business, professional, and political leaders—if they pay attention to the science and technology exploding around them. It is a chapter, says its author, "about health care leadership in an age of scientific advance," and it may well be the most vital chapter in this book.

Nevertheless, I could not resist the temptation to have the last word in the form of an epilogue (chapter 13) on the notion of progress.

References

1. Peter Schwartz, *The Art of the Long View: Paths to Strategic Insight for Yourself and Your Company* (New York: Currency/Doubleday, 1996), p. 166.

2. John Naisbitt, *Megatrends: Ten New Directions Transforming Our Lives* (New York: Warner Books, 1984).

3. Diane Coyle, *The Weightless World: Strategies for Managing the Digital Economy* (Cambridge, MA: The MIT Press, 1998), p. 96.

4. Ibid., p. 144.

5. Ibid., p. 148.

6. Nancy A. Kreider and B. J. Haselton, eds., *The Systems Challenge: Getting the Clinical Information Support You Need to Improve Patient Care* (Chicago: AHA Press, 1997).

7. Roy Ziegler, ed., *Change Drivers: Information Systems for Managed Care* (Chicago: AHA Press, 1998), p. xi.

8. Ibid., p. xvi.

TRENDS
IN TECHNOLOGY

CHAPTER 1

THE RATE OF CHANGE

Within the lifetime of an American physician born in 1827,

local transportation changed from virtually the "hoof and sail"
methods in use in the time of Homer; grain ceased to be cut in
the state by thrusting the sickle into the ripened grain as in the
days of Ruth and threshing done by trampling out by horses on
the threshing-floor or by flail; getting a living and making a
home ceased to be conducted under one roof by the majority of
the American people; education ceased to be a luxury accessible only to the few; in his own field of medicine the X-ray, anesthetics, asepsis, and other developments tended to make the
healing art a science; electricity, the telephone, telegraph and
radio appeared; and the theory of evolution shook the theolog-
ical cosmogony that had reigned for centuries.[1]

Robert and Helen Lynd's classic sociological study of middle America, *Middletown*, from which this passage is derived, was published
less than 70 years ago. It does not mention television, virtual reality,
nuclear power, genetic engineering, holographics, space travel, quantum mechanics, computers, robots, CAT scanners, or automatic cat lit-
ter boxes, to name just a few of the technological marvels of the past
few decades.

ANTICIPATING CHANGE

To the Lynds, as to most other folks in the 1920s, radio, the telephone,
and the automobile were marvelous enough. My own family did not

acquire its first TV, with a nine-inch monochrome screen, until about 1952. Aldous Huxley's classic *Brave New World*, written in 1932, seemed to go way out on a limb at the time in putting a TV set at the end of every bed in a hospital several hundred years into the future.[2] The Lynds, Huxley, and others have studied change but have had a tendency to underestimate the *acceleration* in the pace of change. In large part, this was because they failed to recognize the messages inherent in the introduction of new technologies.

In a 1998 joint press conference with British Prime Minister Tony Blair, President Clinton said that the faster the pace of change, the further into the future it becomes necessary to look.[3] It is necessary because the accelerating pace of demographic, technological, economic, political, and social change causes uncertainty, information overload, and difficulty in making (or reluctance to make) long-term plans. In health care, as in every other field, it is imperative to conduct research to identify the significant trends, inform people of the results of the research, and be prepared not just *for* change but also *to* change, philosophically and pragmatically; all the while maintaining stability in the health care system and not losing focus on its core values. This in turn implies the incorporation of futures issues in continuing medical education and providing students (who include practitioners) with the technology and training to filter relevant information from the flood.

Then the question is: How far ahead do we need to look? In today's turbulent health care sector, it seems hard enough to look just a year or two ahead. Managed care consultant Roy Ziegler's recent AHA Press book *Change Drivers* takes health care leaders through the immediate challenges of what he calls "a *rapidly changing* marketplace" in which "information systems are being dismantled and reengineered *at breakneck speed*" (emphasis added).[4] These phrases are not hyperbole. The first 80 years of the twentieth century were a continuation of the comfortable pace of fee-for-service health care, with relatively minor incremental improvements in the paper-based information systems on which it relied. The following 15 years saw the health maintenance organization (HMO), supported by the rapid computerization of information systems, sweep much of fee-for-service under the rug of history, and the past five years have seen the accelerated evolutionary morphing of the HMO paradigm into managed care, integrated delivery systems, and other variants.

The acceleration in the spread of computers, the Internet, medical information bases such as Medline, and even the contents of the doctor's black bag (such as cheap electronic blood pressure monitors) among not just providers but patients as well portends more morphing in the first few years of the twenty-first century toward a paradigm in which patients assume greater responsibility for their own health care management. But as we shall see, it does not stop there. As Ziegler says, "It is not simply that non-information systems managers and executives will have to acquire a rudimentary level of computer literacy. The challenge is more profound: They will have to become accustomed to, and learn to shape and direct, the constant change fostered by the rapid evolution of information technology."[5]

Non-IS (information systems) managers and executives need not be too concerned about the need to acquire computer literacy—not in the time scale with which this book is concerned. I shall show that well within 30 years the computer will have acquired much more than a rudimentary level of "people literacy" and will have become invisible *as* a "computer."

In this book, we focus on change in the business and practice of health care. But that change is not occurring in a vacuum; the forces of change operating on health care are also at work in the wider domains of economics, politics, and society. The forces are primarily technological. In fact, I believe most major change throughout human history has been due to changes in technology, and particularly to changes in the technologies of communication.

For roughly the first million years of human existence, there were no technologies of communication. Even spoken language (which, relying on no external artifacts, does not count as a technology) may only have arisen in the past 100,000 years or less. The first communication technology—*writing*—appeared in Sumeria about 6,000 years ago.[6] Writing put control of information—and therefore, ultimately, of people—into the hands of those few who could master it or who could afford to employ the scribes who could master it. Writing ended aeons of bottom-up oral tradition binding family and tribal society through the open and largely indiscriminate sharing of information and started 3,000 years of top-down feudalism, in which information (and power) became concentrated in documents that discriminated between the few who could read and the many who could not.

The second major technology, *printing*, gave more people access to much the same information their kings and barons possessed. As

Marshall McLuhan remarked, it turned everyone into a reader.[7] Over the course of five centuries, the printing press virtually destroyed feudalism and fostered early forms of democracy. The American Revolution was as much a product of the printed revolutionary pamphlet as it was of American courage and British political incompetence.

The *broadcasting* technologies of radio and (especially) TV brought more information to more people more quickly. The copy machine and the sound cassette recorder—*narrowcasting devices* each representing personal forms of the print and broadcast media—allowed people to turn from being readers—receivers of information—into publishers (McLuhan). They gave revolutionaries the means to sidestep state control of broadcast and print media.

Every major advance in information technology has had an historic revolutionary impact on society.[8] Each has produced a shift in the social paradigm, ending the status quo and taking society in unanticipated new directions. When change occurs slowly over millennia, as in the case of writing, or over centuries, as in the case of printing, then there is no perceived importance to anticipating it. But when change is likely to occur within our lifetime or within the span of our professional career, then we *must* pay attention.

Most political, business, educational, and social leaders and researchers were caught flat-footed by the hippie movement, women's liberation, gay rights, and other technology-enhanced phenomena of the 1960s. They now recognize that change, at all levels of organization, is an inevitable and increasingly rapid consequence of the introduction of new information technologies and communication media and that they must therefore anticipate and be prepared to embrace the new technologies in order to have at least some semblance of control over the rate and direction of change.

The problem lies in knowing what to anticipate. One of the great failures of our age has been that of academia to explain and predict social change, with rare exceptions such as McLuhan (whose insights were largely discounted by his contemporary fellow academicians). This is one reason why some political and business leaders have turned to a distinctly unacademic group to help them get a handle on the future—science fiction writers.

Political leaders from Theodore Roosevelt to Ronald Reagan and businesses from Microsoft to Finland's telecommunications giant Nokia have consulted with science fiction writers, and there is a steady but discreet trade in high-level corporate and government consultancy for the better-known writers.[9] Science fiction seems somehow disreputable; while one must take occasional solace there, one ought not to be seen openly in its company.

In this final year of the second millennium, we are already several decades into the evolution of another major new information technology: computerized networking. Like its predecessor technologies of writing, printing, broadcasting, and narrowcasting, computerized networking is forcing major change on society and its components, including the health care component—not only because it represents an amalgamation of all previous communication technologies (in many ways returning us to the pretechnology era of oral tradition), but also because it introduces a third party into the processes of information storage, manipulation, and communication. *The third party is a machine.*

In the early 1990s the main mediation role played by the computer in human-human communications was in assembling and routing packets of information so they reached their intended recipient. There was always a human being at the sending and receiving ends of any communication. But today the computer plays a bigger, more powerful, and increasingly autonomous role through software robots that can decide what we read and where we go on the Web. They talk among themselves, do some of our thinking for us, and are literally evolving—at an accelerating rate.

The most recent technologies of computing, the Internet, robotics, and artificial intelligence convey two messages: (1) machines are evolving toward some form of life, and (2) our own individual capabilities are being extended. The first message is highly contentious and the subject of another book, but the second is particularly relevant to a health care system that recognizes patient self-care as a desirable feature of demand management because the technologies are extending the individual's self-care capabilities.

In retrospect, the impetus for the accelerated development of these modern technologies is not hard to find. Computers have demonstrably driven technology development, and technology has fed back to drive computer development. For example, computers have helped design micromanufacturing technology that, in turn, has helped create denser and therefore more powerful computers. For another example, computers led to the development of the Internet, and the Internet in turn is driving the development of more powerful hardware and software.

Because it is a recursive process fueled by an inexhaustible energy supply (bits of information, or what biologist Richard Dawkins has termed *memes*[10]), the acceleration of change in technology is *exponential*. Few people appear to have grasped the full significance of this, perhaps because up to this point in history the rise in the acceleration curve has been shallow enough, and our individual minds and collective cultures have been adaptive enough, that we have had time to adjust to the changes wrought by the introduction of new technologies but not enough time to consider their full implications.

THE ACCELERATION CURVE

If we are to help our business, economic, political, and health care leaders to anticipate the implications of, and have some control over, change, then we need first to determine the acceleration curve prospectively and not merely retrospectively. As a concept, "change" cannot be measured, but change to the definable components of a process or thing even as broad as health care can be measured indirectly using the acceleration in the growth of the power of computers and the Internet—the technologies at the heart of the growth in medical and other technologies.

The measure of acceleration in computing power is supplied by "Moore's law," formulated by Intel cofounder Gordon Moore in 1965. Formally, it asserts that the number of elements in advanced integrated circuits doubles every 18 to 24 months.[11] Informally, it is commonly interpreted to mean that computer performance doubles every 18 months.

The general truth of Moore's law can be perceived first in figure 1-1, showing the introduction of the various generations of Intel chips; and second in my adaptation (figure 1-2) of a graph from roboticist Hans Moravec's book *Mind Children*.[12] It substantiates Moore's law up to 1988 and predicts an acceleration in computing power such that by the year 2030 we will be using $1,000 desktop (or palmtop or implanted) computers, each as powerful in processing capacity and memory storage as current estimates of the human brain.

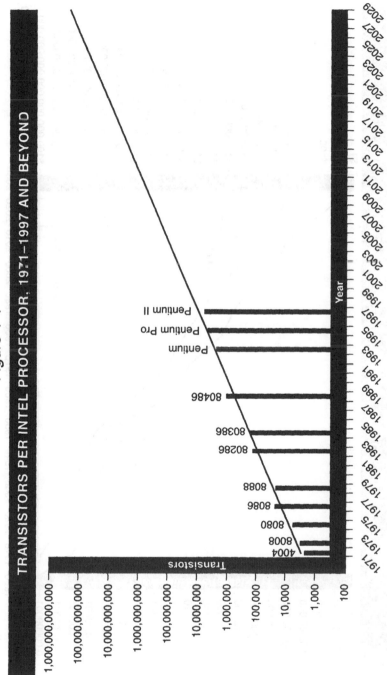

Figure 1-1

TRANSISTORS PER INTEL PROCESSOR, 1971–1997 AND BEYOND

Data from Intel Web site at http://www.intel.com/Intel/museum/25anniv/hot1specs.ht.

Figure 1-2

GROWING POWER AND FALLING COST OF COMPUTING

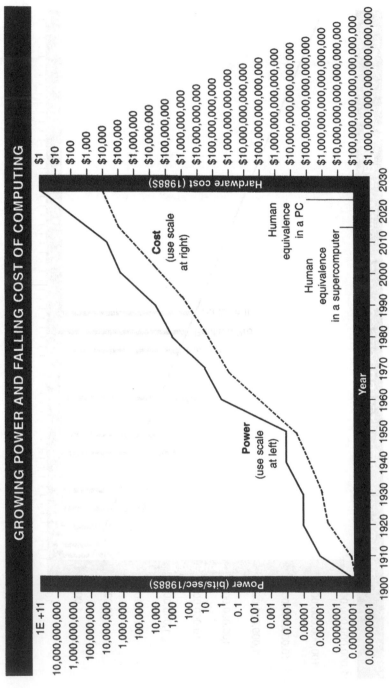

Adapted from Hans Moravec, Mind Children: The Future of Robot and Human Intelligence (Cambridge, MA: Harvard University Press, 1988), p. 64.

Bob Metcalfe, creator of the Ethernet LAN protocol, is credited with a macrocosmic corollary to Moore's microcosmic law. "Metcalfe's law" holds that the value of networks rises by the square of the power of all the computers attached to them.[13] This is vague compared to Moore's law, absent definitions of "value" and "power," but few who use networks would disagree that they grow more "valuable" as they grow larger, assuming reliability, robustness, and speed.

We tend to think of a network as a group of individual computers linked through cables at distances ranging from a few feet in the case of LANs (local-area networks) to thousands of miles in the case of WANs (wide-area networks, of which the Internet is the ultimate expression). But it is important to note, as we shall see in the next chapter, that an individual computer can itself be a network of internal processors—little computers—linked over distances measured in millimeters.

Today, there are relatively few isolated networks. Most LANs, and therefore the computers attached to them, have been essentially tied together to form one vast global network—the Internet. Figures 1-3a and 1-3b show the exponential growth in (1) the number of computers, known as *hosts*, which provide some sort of service or function on the Internet (such as a mail, news, or Web server),[14] and (2) the speed of the connections linking the host computers to one another and to your desktop. This speed is known as *bandwidth*, and the chart traces growth in Internet backbone (the central artery through which tributary arteries are interlinked) and user (tributary) bandwidth.[15] The growth in both backbone and user bandwidth is accelerating even more exponentially than the growth in hosts. This has particular significance in the context of health care because telemedicine—a rapidly evolving set of technologies we shall examine in later chapters—requires very high bandwidth for the transmission of high-resolution images, including not just today's x-rays and videoconferences but also tomorrow's three-dimensional haptic holograms of patients undergoing telesurgery.

GENERALIZING THE RATE OF CHANGE

Recalling that this book sets out to look some 30 years into the future, it seems reasonable, if only on the basis of the forgoing evidence and the continuing upward thrust of the trend lines shown in the graphs, to conclude that Moore's and Metcalfe's laws, in their popular interpretation

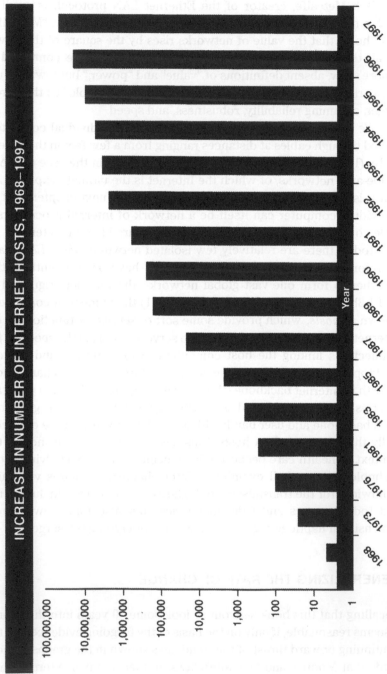

Figure 1-3a

INCREASE IN NUMBER OF INTERNET HOSTS, 1968–1997

Year

100,000,000
10,000,000
1,000,000
100,000
10,000
1,000
100
10
1

1968 1973 1976 1981 1983 1985 1987 1989 1990 1991 1992 1993 1994 1995 1996 1997

Data from ftp://nic.merit.edu/nsfnet/statistics/history.hosts.

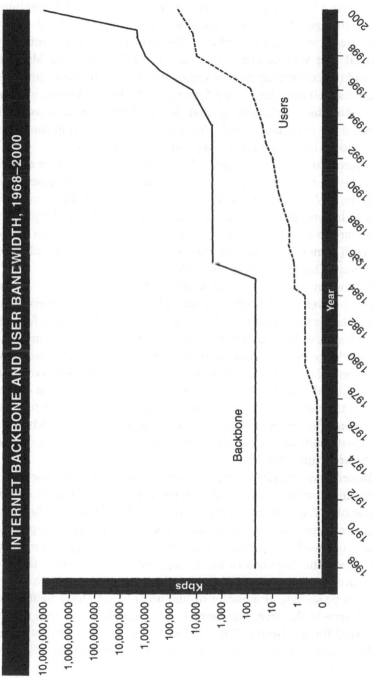

Figure 1-3b

INTERNET BACKBONE AND USER BANDWIDTH, 1968–2000

Backbone data partly from Vinton Cerf's September 1997 paper "Beyond the Millennium: The Internet," http://www.mci.com/mcisearch/aboutyou/interests/technology/ontech/cerfreport0897.shtml.

as measures of growth in computer and network power, will continue to operate through 2029 as they have since they were formulated. Chapter 2 will present evidence of technologies already developed but not yet deployed that will maintain the validity of Moore's and Metcalfe's laws and the continuing upward exponential thrust of the trend lines in the graphs well into the twenty-first century. (There is some evidence, as we shall see in chapter 2, that Moore himself may have underestimated the exponent, in which case the acceleration in the pace of change could be even greater than posited in this book.)

Moore's law was formulated in 1965. From 1965 to 2029 is a total of 64 years—the number of squares on a chessboard. The Chinese are said to tell the fable of a eunuch who asked, as a reward for services rendered to his emperor, for a single grain of rice on the first square of a chessboard to be successively doubled on the second through the 64th squares. The nonmathematical emperor laughingly agreed, only to discover that he had given away more than all the rice in China.

A modern analogy to this story is that humanity has awarded computer-driven technology with bits of knowledge at 100 percent compound interest per annum. At that rate, it cannot take long before technology knows at least as much as we do, even though the sum total of our knowledge may seem astronomical in terms of bits. The next chapter presents the evidence that Moore's and Metcalfe's laws have already been validated and that we have been paying interest and will continue to do so through the year 2030 and beyond. The evidence is presented in the form of a description of current developments and trends in technologies that are sure to be introduced into the business and practice of health care within 30 years.

Moore's law is a rare example of a successful attempt to predict the future, and computer chip maker Intel, for one, has staked and won billions of dollars on its validity and reliability. Similarly, Sun Microcomputer Corporation seems to have based its winning strategy of selling network-ready servers and workstations—a strategy summed up in the slogan "The Network *Is* the Computer"—on Metcalfe's law. Such "laws" are not like the laws of physics, nor even like scientific theories. They can be shown, as a matter of historical fact, to have held approximately true in the past, but there is no scientific proof that they will hold good for the future. They are more like working hypotheses or applied common sense: reasonable rules of thumb that are neither certain nor precise.

Rules of thumb are more common in science, engineering, and medicine than most people realize. The reason is simple: They seem to work, they have been right so far, and, in the absence of anything better, they must still be presumed to point in the direction of truth even if their accuracy is suspect at some arbitrary level of detail.

References and Notes

1. Robert Lynd and Helen Lynd, *Middletown: A Study in American Culture* (New York: Harcourt Brace Jovanovich, 1929).

2. Aldous Huxley, *Brave New World & Brave New World Revisited* (New York: Harper Collins, 1960). *Brave New World* originally published in 1932.

3. His words were: "In a funny way, when societies change as fast and as much as our societies are changing today, when the pace of events and their variety make it more difficult to predict what will happen next week or next month, it is even more important to be oriented toward the long term, because you have to figure that if you lay in a structure of opportunity for a free people, they'll get it right and they'll overcome all these unpredictable developments in the meanwhile." Transcript of press conference at http://library.whitehouse.gov/.

4. Roy Ziegler, ed., *Change Drivers: Information Systems for Managed Care* (Chicago: AHA Press, 1998), pp. xi, xiii.

5. Ibid., p. xvi.

6. See Everett M. Rogers, *Communication Technology: The New Media in Society* (New York: The Free Press, 1986), p. 27.

7. See Philip Marchand, *Marshall McLuhan: The Medium and the Messenger* (Cambridge, MA: The MIT Press, 1998), p. 273.

8. Marshall McLuhan was one of the first to recognize and predict the effects of the broadcast media on society, but for a more retrospective (and therefore better-informed) and more readable analysis of those effects, see Joshua Meyrowitz, *No Sense of Place: The Impact of Electronic Media on Social Behavior* (New York: Oxford University Press, 1985).

9. Elizabeth Wiese, "Firms Look To Sci-Fi Writers For Advice," *USA Today* (July 22, 1998). Franklin Delano Roosevelt met with H. G. Wells in 1906; a bevy of science fiction writers participated in President Reagan's Strategic Defense Initiative ("Star Wars") advisory panel; Nokia commissioned such luminaries as Arthur C. Clarke and Nicholas Negroponte to write future predictive articles for a book published privately within the company.

10. See Richard Dawkins, *The Selfish Gene* (Oxford, UK: Oxford University Press, 1976).

11. For an update from the horse's mouth, see "An Update on Moore's Law" at http://www2.intel.com/pressroom/archive/speeches/gem93 097.htm.

12. Hans Moravec, *Mind Children: The Future of Robot and Human Intelligence* (Cambridge, MA: Harvard University Press, 1988).

13. Strictly speaking, the law was coined by George Gilder—who credited Metcalfe with the idea behind it—in an article published in *Forbes ASAP* (September 13, 1993). The article is online at http://www.forbes.com/asap/gilder/telecosm4a.htm.

14. Data from ftp://nic.merit.edu/nsfnet/statistics/history.hosts.

15. Backbone data partly from Vinton Cerf's September 1997 paper "Beyond the Millennium: The Internet," http://www.mci.com/mci search/aboutyou/interests/technology/ontech/cerfreport0897.shtml; user data represent the commercial introduction of telephone and cable modems from 110 bps through 10 Mbps (existing) and 43 Mbps (under development at Zenith).

CHAPTER 2

FUNDAMENTAL TRENDS
IN TECHNOLOGY

A turn-of-the millennium stroll through almost any modern medical facility will surely reveal a broad array of technologies. Receptionists and clerks punch patient information and doctors' appointments into networked PCs. Some physicians may be seen making their rounds muttering observations not to an accompanying nurse but to a cassette recorder. Some are even talking into computerized speech-recognition devices that not only record but also transcribe. In the wards, patient beds may be festooned with catheters, automatic drug-dispensing devices, and various monitors, not to mention TVs and telephones. In the labs and operating theaters, data displays and moving graphs glow greenly amidst dials and switches and cables and tubes, and space age scanners crowd out the quaint x-ray machine. Buried in the bowels of all these devices lies a computer chip.

Oh, and by the way, nurses are outnumbered by auxiliaries.

This is a far cry from 30 years ago, when the CAT scanner had not yet been invented, x-rays and EKGs ruled the labs and theaters, the typewriter ran the desktop, and matron commanded the wards. Thirty years from now, as a result of the acceleration in the pace of change we analyzed in chapter 1, the picture will be just as dramatically different. There will be few wards and few medical facilities as we know them today. Much of the technology of care will have been transferred to individual homes. And doctors, nurses, and auxiliaries will be outnumbered by intelligent robots.

This may seem a fanciful scenario, but in this chapter I intend to show that by the year 2030 we will be awash in computing power of cosmic proportions, and this power will be the basis for the following:

- Intelligent subminiature drug and tissue manufacturing machine processes that can be implanted in the body to perform medical and surgical tasks
- Autonomous mobile robots driven by software and possessing more than human levels of intelligence, at least in specific domains of knowledge and expertise, as well as superhuman sensory perception and manipulative capabilities
- Workplaces, including doctors' offices and clinics, that exist only in virtual reality
- The interconnection of all these new artifacts through a vastly improved Internet, enabling them to remotely monitor, troubleshoot, repair, augment, and improve one another, share information with one another and with us, gather and analyze data on a vast scale, and act on them
- The emergence out of this uncontrollable intelligent network of something wholly new, advanced, and unexpected

Some 20 key technologies, grouped into functional classifications as shown in figure 2-1, are already widely deployed in various parts of the health care system, and trends in their development can therefore be expected to influence the system's future.

In this and subsequent chapters, I present an overview of what each particular technology is, illustrate by means of real-world examples what it can do today in practice or in the research lab, and forecast what it is predicted to do over the next 30 years—a period well within the lifetimes of many of the readers of this book.

The base of the pyramid—the architectures of computing—is the essential support for the hardware and software engines that already control the technologies used in health care, and it is on the base and the second tier that we shall focus in this chapter. The stronger the base, the "heavier" can be the structures it supports. We begin by describing just how much stronger the base will grow over the next 30 years. The subject of computing is not as remote from the interests of the intended audience for this book as it may first seem, and the reader—technically oriented or not—is urged not to skip over it.

Figure 2-1

PYRAMID OF HEALTH CARE TECHNOLOGIES

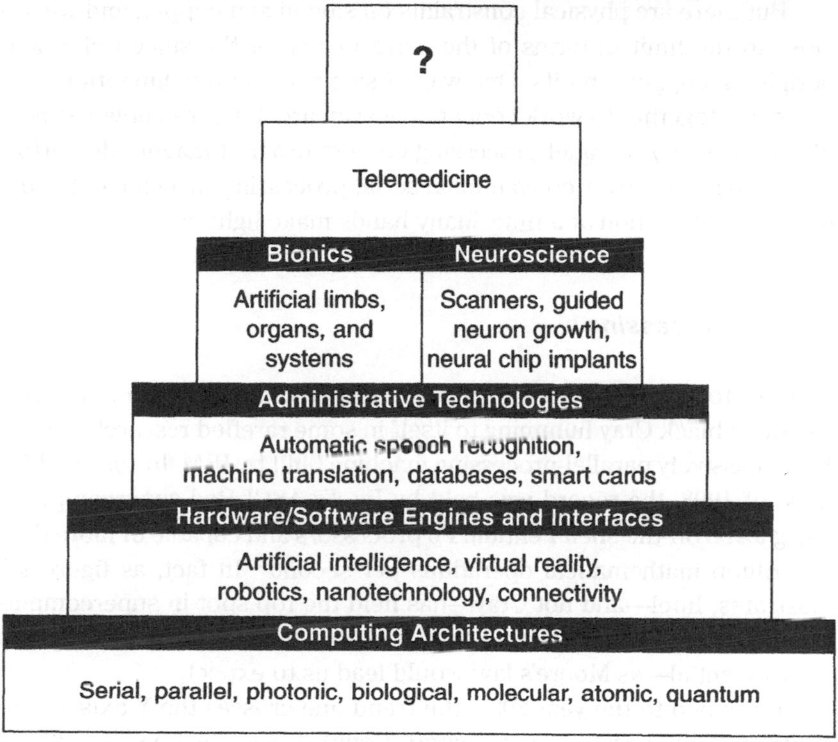

?

Telemedicine

Bionics	Neuroscience
Artificial limbs, organs, and systems	Scanners, guided neuron growth, neural chip implants

Administrative Technologies

Automatic speech recognition, machine translation, databases, smart cards

Hardware/Software Engines and Interfaces

Artificial intelligence, virtual reality, robotics, nanotechnology, connectivity

Computing Architectures

Serial, parallel, photonic, biological, molecular, atomic, quantum

TRENDS IN COMPUTING ARCHITECTURES

When Moore's law bumps up against the constraints of the real laws of physics, the ultimate power of a computer is determined by the architecture of the chip—what materials it is made from and how the building blocks are arranged and connected. The serial PC you are using today has gone through exponential jumps in performance through the use of new building blocks—from vacuum tube through transistor to integrated silicon circuit.

Gordon Moore's colleague and chief operating officer at Intel, Craig Barrett, said in 1997 that the capabilities found in the $50,000 to $75,000 workstations that produced the animations for the movie *Jurassic Park* would soon be available in $2,000 PCs, and that PCs in the year 2011 would use a billion-transistor chip, compared with about 8 million in the most advanced Pentium chip in 1997.[1]

But there are physical constraints on silicon and copper, and we are close to the limit in terms of the performance of the silicon chip and peripheral copper circuits. One way of sidestepping this limitation is to link chips together to work cooperatively; an architecture known as *parallel processing*. Parallel processing confers order-of-magnitude performance increases over conventional serial processing, which can handle only one calculation at a time. Many hands make light work.

Parallel Processing

As of October 1998, the world's fastest supercomputer was no longer a gleaming black Cray humming to itself in some rarefied research citadel, but a massively parallel-processing machine built by IBM. In 1997 and for most of 1998, the record was held by Intel's ASCI Red supercomputer, using 9,152 off-the-shelf Pentium P6 processors and capable of more than 1.3 trillion mathematical operations per second.[2] In fact, as figure 2-2 illustrates, Intel—and not Cray—has held the top spot in supercomputing for nearly all of the 1990s.[3] Note, too, that the trend line of the graph is exponential—as Moore's law would lead us to expect.

Extended to the year 2030, the trend line crosses the Y axis at 10^{22} floating point operations per second (flops). Ten to the power of 22 is a quantity so rare scientists have not bothered to name it. The largest scientific prefix for an exponent is *exa*, or 10^{18}. Our number is 10 thousand times bigger than an exaflop.

But IBM is already set to beat its own record. In February 1998 IBM signed an $85 million contract with the Department of Energy and the Lawrence Livermore National Laboratory to deliver in the year 2000 a parallel-processing supercomputer system capable of 10 trillion calculations per second.[4] The computer will calculate in a single second what would take 10 million years using a handheld calculator. It represents an eightfold increase in simulation detail compared to what was available in 1998. Yet Moore's law would predict a "mere" 5.2 trillion-calculations-per-second machine in 2000. The balance can probably be accounted for by the synergy between Moore's and Metcalfe's laws in parallel processing.

Figure 2-2

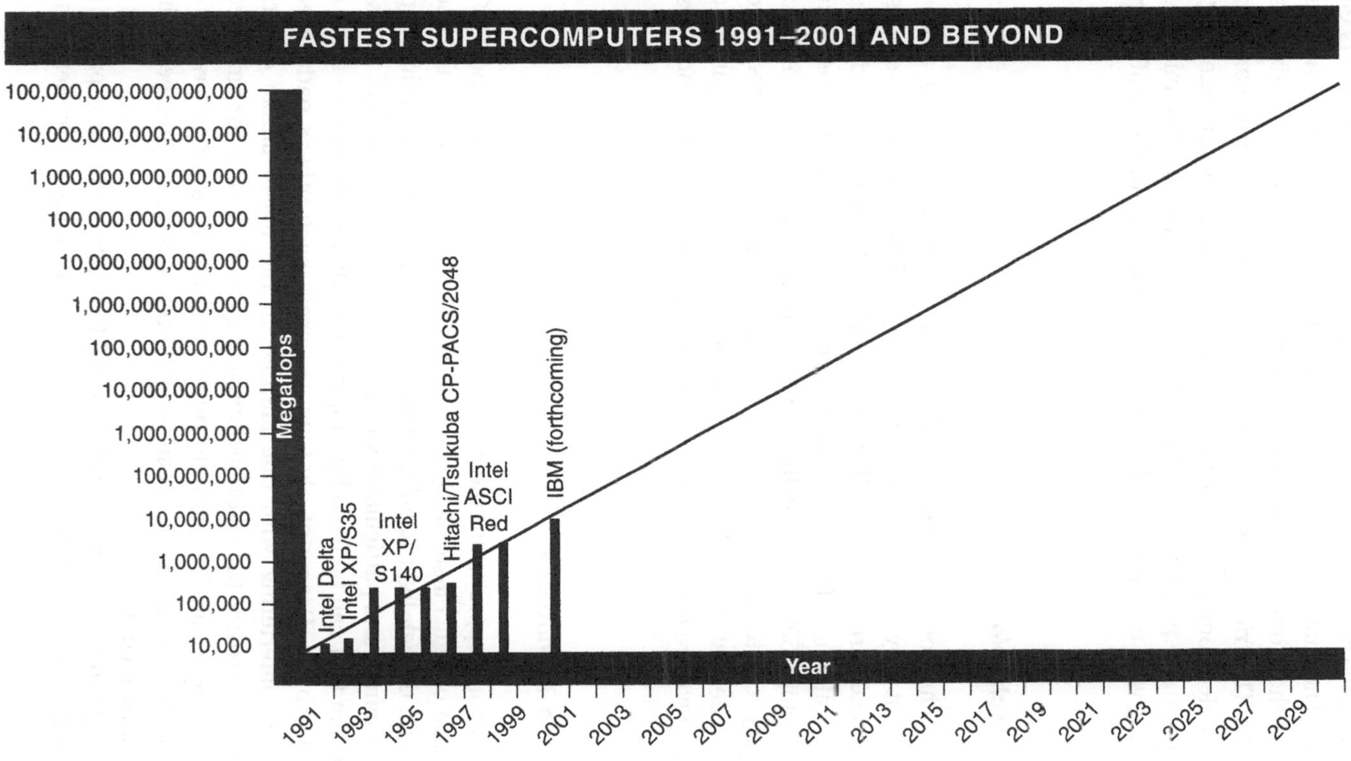

FASTEST SUPERCOMPUTERS 1991–2001 AND BEYOND

Data from Top 500 Supercomputers Web site at http://www.netlib.org/benchmark/top500/top500.list.html.

21

But physical constraints remain as long as the architecture is electronic. The main constraint is the speed of the electron, which rubs against the atoms of its carrier and slows to a thousandth of the speed of light. The friction also causes heat. Worst of all, electrons are sensitive to electromagnetic interference. Two approaches are emerging to counter these problems. The first uses *nanotechnology*—techniques for working with materials (such as individual atoms) a billionth of a meter in size.

Nanotechnology

Nanotechnologists cannot yet build materials or machines atom by atom, but they have succeeded in building carbon nanotubes—sheets of hexagonal carbon atoms rolled into cylinders. Nanotubes could be used to etch silicon at finer scales than current laser-etching devices (resulting in chips 500 times smaller than a Pentium) and to perform microsurgery on tissue as small as an individual cell. Nanotechnology researchers at NASA, IBM, and other leading technology organizations believe we are only "three to five years" away from seeing nanotubes in practical use.[5]

Photon Technology

The second approach to the electron problem is to use the photon (the particle of light) instead. By definition, the photon travels at the speed of light, though light itself is slowed down in anything less than a perfect vacuum and particularly when constrained within optical fibers—a problem that can be fixed by "doping" the fiber with the rare earth element erbium. Beams of photons can cross each other's path directly without interfering with one another in the least—unlike electrical wires. To provide the on-off switches or gates necessary for binary computing, miniscule holographic representations of a prism—which can bend light just like a real prism—can be generated (at lightspeed) within the optical circuits.

A photonic chip was built by AT&T Bell Labs in the early part of this decade,[6] but major research has not been pursued because there remain some "hard" (which means expensive, not impossible) problems to solve and because it has so far been more economical to incrementally improve the performance of electronic chips than to create photonic ones. But as the physical limits of electronic computers are approached and the complexity of parallel circuitry becomes too great to manage, we can expect a renewed research effort on photonic computers—unless another nonelectronic approach proves more feasible. Besides photonic computing, other nonelectronic approaches include using the computing capabilities of genetically engineered bacteria, atoms, and the extraordinary properties of subatomic particles.

Other Nonelectronic Approaches

A type of bacteria commonly found in the San Francisco Bay coastal marshes owes its purple color to the bacteriarhodopsin (bR) protein, which converts photons into cellular energy. Devices made with bR can be constructed that will switch between alternate on-off states when bathed in red and green laser light. Thus, the bacteria can be induced to perform binary logic. Such devices would operate thousands of time faster than electronic computers, might be much less expensive than photonic computers, and would provide massively parallel and massively distributed processing capabilities in a computer that would fit in your shirt pocket.[7]

The scanning tunneling microscope, originally designed to look at atoms, can also be used to manipulate atoms and use them to compute. Such a device could offer tens to hundreds of terabytes of information storage capacity and fit inside a standard CD-ROM drive. Even smaller than the atom are the subatomic particles, or *quanta*, considered to be the basic building blocks of matter. Quantum computing takes advantage of the fact that subatomic particles, unobserved, occupy multiple states all at once. Instead of being on or off, left or right, up or down, they are on and off, left and right, up and down—simultaneously.

Two methods have been used to get quanta to compute without being observed (which would ruin the computation). One involves trapping a single particle and cooling it to just slightly above absolute zero—a tricky and costly process, but it has been done. The other uses the statistical properties of trillions of trillions of quanta in a thermal ensemble such as a cup of coffee, where it doesn't matter statistically if a few trillion particles are observed.[8] Because of the multiple states of quanta, they can be used as logic gates with multiple or "qubit" (quantum bit) states—not just the binary on-off states of conventional logic gates—which produce a combinatorial explosion of processing power. The details of how it works need not concern us; our focus is on the power of such mechanisms. To factor a 1,000-digit number would take the Intel ASCI Red longer than the estimated 100 billion years of life left for the universe. A quantum computer would do it "while-u-wait."

In 1997 scientists demonstrated a quantum computer that could add 2 plus 2. Not much, but—as the eunuch said to the emperor—it's a start. A year later, researchers at Yale University created a single-electron transistor that could lead to the development of quantum computers the size of a thumbtack with supercomputer powers.[9]

All of these devices face a daunting learning and manufacturing curve and are at least 10 to 15 years away from production. This coincides with current estimates of the life remaining for conventional semiconductors, as the fabrication plant costs for multibillion-transistor chips will by then approach the GNP of the planet (a new Intel plant announced in February 1998 had a price tag of $1.5 billion). Biomolecular computers offer the promise of being economically grown in a vat for a few million dollars, versus the billion dollar costs of today's Intel and IBM chip fabrication plants. Quantum computers could eventually cost little more than a cup of coffee.

It bears stressing that none of these devices is theoretical, still less science fiction. Photonic, molecular, and quantum computers have all been demonstrated to work, and the only issue is the current cost of R&D and manufacturing.

FORECAST: By the year 2030, we will be awash in computing power of cosmic proportions.

That power will reside in the hardware and software engines and interfaces that drive health care technologies. The next section discusses trends in the engines and interfaces.

KEY TRENDS IN HARDWARE AND SOFTWARE
ENGINES AND INTERFACES

The following eight key features are visible trends in the ongoing development of hardware, software, and the ways in which we interact with them:

1. Smart
2. Small
3. Mobile and dextrous
4. Aware
5. Communicative
6. Interconnected
7. Autonomous
8. Complex

Each of these features individually promises to have a revolutionary impact on medicine.

Smart

First, software is getting smarter through artificial intelligence (AI). Much of the recent breakthrough development in AI has resulted from the integration of rule-based *expert systems* that operate strictly algorithmically (if exactly this, then exactly that) with fuzzy connectionist systems called *neural networks* that operate heuristically (on rules of thumb—if approximately this, then probably that). As a result, computers now think more like humans and less like computers.

Already we have AI programs that can beat the World Chess Grandmaster at his own game, expertly diagnose pain, identify abnormal EKGs and diagnose heart attacks better than cardiologists, detect Pap smear abnormalities better than cytologists, and screen mammograms for signs of breast cancer more efficiently and effectively than radiologists. Specific companies producing these products and services as of late 1998 are listed below. (Endnotes provide links to further information.)

- A company called NovaTelligence is selling a PC-based expert system for the diagnosis of acute and chronic pain. PMA (Pain

Management Advisor) embodies the expertise of noted pain specialists Dr. Mark Wallace of the University of California, San Diego School of Medicine, and Dr. Gordon Irving of the University of Texas Medical School at Houston. The PMA system contains all currently available pain treatment algorithms and modalities.[10]

- *Circulation*, journal of the American Heart Association, has reported that an AI program combining neural net technology with expert-system technology did better than a group of cardiologists in diagnosing heart attacks and was 10 percent better at identifying abnormal EKGs than the most experienced cardiologist.[11]

- PAPNET, a neural network program, increases the accuracy of cervical screening by analyzing Pap smears and displaying potentially abnormal cells for review and analysis by a cytology professional. In tests, even after manual double-screening of Pap smears, PAPNET detected significant numbers of previously undetected abnormalities.[12] The Royal Liverpool University Hospital became the first U.K. National Health Service cervical screening center to use PAPNET.[13]

- World Chess Grandmaster Garry Kasparov was beaten by an AI-driven computer in early 1998. There is a level of complexity in chess beyond which even Kasparov's brain cannot go, but AI-driven machines with sufficient power can, and Moore's law last year supplied sufficient power.

- Network-savvy AI software modules, called *intelligent agents* or *softbots* (software robots) or just *bots*, prepare individually customized online newspapers for millions of Internet users. Bots work faster, more efficiently, and at much less cost than humans.[14]

- Bots also act as Internet postmasters, network administrators and troubleshooters, and someone to talk with—including a Rogerian psychotherapist so dumb it fools many people into thinking it is human.

- Medicaid in Texas is being turned over to AI "policebots," already successfully used by telephone and credit card companies to detect and prevent fraud. Policebots are more effective, efficient, reliable, and trustworthy than people in this role and, of course, less expensive.[15]

- A NASA shuttle scheduled to fly this year will have something approaching the HAL of Stanley Kubrick and Arthur C. Clarke's *2001* science fiction movie. NASA calls it dMARS, a collection of softbots capable of monitoring a shuttle (and ultimately the planned space station) and its crew and making decisions.[16]

- Some mortgage lenders are now using AI software to prescreen loan applicants, and a British company has just begun selling a neural net software package for assessing a bank or mortgage customer's creditworthiness. In trials with some 20 banks, the program outperformed human loan officers, achieving an average reduction in bad debt of 10 percent while increasing the number of applicants accepted.[17]
- The computer game version of the movie *Blade Runner* includes 70 characters, each endowed with their own individual AI, against whom the human player must match wits.[18] One PC-based flight simulator has hundreds of warplanes fighting their own battles while the human player-pilot tries to fit in.[19]

FORECAST: By the year 2030, software will have developed domain-specific intelligence, knowledge, and expertise of at least equivalent capability to most low- and middle-level and some top-level white-collar workers in all industries and professions, including the medical and nursing professions.

Small

Hardware is getting smaller through developments in miniaturization and its extreme expression, *nanotechnology*, which we met briefly in discussing the application of nanotubes in computer chip manufacturing and microsurgery. Nanotechnology is technology for building things—ultimately, anything—atom by atom and molecule by molecule. The molecular and atomic computers mentioned earlier are examples of nanoscale (billionths of a meter) devices.

Nanotechnologists hope to build nanoscale devices called *universal assemblers* that can reconfigure their environment into something else, molecule by molecule. Instead of an entertainment center loaded with music CD player, DVD player, TV set, radio, VCR, and so on, you would have a single device made up of trillions of universal assemblers that could, at your command, reconfigure a TV set into a radio, a VCR, or even a perfect reproduction of the Mona Lisa.

One company, Zyvex, is on the road to building such a device.[20] In late 1998, Zyvex and Washington University demonstrated one key component of a universal assembler: a nanomanipulator to manipulate atoms or the carbon nanotubes that have such exciting implications for surgery (among many other things). Zyvex's nanomanipulator is much more precise than the scanning tunneling microscope method used by IBM researchers to build the letters "IBM" out of a few atoms.

The company's founder and CEO said he has no illusions about the enormity of his company's undertaking. He estimates it will take Zyvex 10 years to build an assembler. What is significant, though, is that investors have not balked at either the difficulties or the time scale involved, and Zyvex has "the people and financing to make it happen."[21]

Meanwhile, at a scale we can at least conceive, Sandia National Laboratories has developed a one-millimeter-square "intelligent" micromachine incorporating computer chip controllers. Such micromachines could be used as tiny drug-delivery devices within the body. By 1995 Sandia had already succeeded in mass-producing micromachines that could perform work—turning gears each one-hundredth the weight of a dust mite at hundreds of thousands of revolutions per minute. Each gear was approximately one-hundredth the thickness of a sheet of paper and smaller in diameter than a human hair.[22]

At nanoscale, of course, things are invisible to the unaided human eye. But technology does not have to be nanoscale to be invisible. Computer chips are routinely built into automobile engines, microwave controls, and even children's dolls, but the chips are not seen unless we take the device apart. This kind of invisibility is a major trend in itself.

A semiphysiotherapeutic application of microminiature devices already deployed in the seats of a luxury-car maker is described in the section below.

> **FORECAST:** By 2030, many light and heavy manufacturing processes will have been replaced by intelligent micro- or nanomanufacturing processes. Such processes may be implanted in the body to perform medical and surgical tasks.

MEMS. Microelectromechanical systems (MEMS) are tiny devices about the width of a human hair. The technology was spun out of research to fabricate integrated circuits on silicon chips and is one of today's fastest-growing technologies. The advantages of a MEMS device over traditional devices are size, weight, power consumption, durability, and cost in large-volume production.

In March 1998 BCAM Technologies Inc.[23] in cooperation with the Microelectronics Center of North Carolina[24] announced a fingernail-sized working prototype of a powerful microvalve using MEMS technology. The valve's airflow rate is an order of magnitude greater than that of any existing microvalve. Traditional valves, including solenoid types, are heavy, power hungry, and expensive.

The microvalve assembly resides on a microchip and is a key component in BCAM's Intelligent Surface Technology (IST) designed for use in any product that comes into contact with the human body, including medical and athletic footwear. An IST system can be made up of several components, including bladders, sensors, a pump, a valve assembly, electronic control circuitry, and software. Of these components, the valve assembly proved a major challenge for microminiaturization.

IST footwear, automobile seats, recliners, bedding, and hand tools can sense and measure the pressure distribution of any part of the body touching their surfaces and then adjust themselves in real time to conform to that particular body, maximizing comfort, fit, and performance and minimizing fatigue and stress. They can also be made to give what BCAM calls "intelligent massage."

The first commercial IST product was introduced in the 1998 Cadillac Seville STS driver and passenger car seats. The online brochure copy reads: "Adaptive seating recognizes individual size and seating position. The seats make an initial adjustment to create a custom fit. A network of 10 air cells and sensors in the seat cushions "read" the seats every four minutes and adjusts for any occupant position changes."[25]

The application of such technology to hospital beds cannot have escaped manufacturers' attention.

Mobile and Dexterous

Machines are becoming more mobile and more dexterous. Mobility is a result of two other trends—miniaturization and intermachine communications. Miniaturization results in computers so small they can be woven into the fabric of garments. The first wearable computer was demonstrated by the MIT Media Lab at a fashion show in 1998.

Increasingly sophisticated methods of wireless communication enable wearable and other embedded computers to stay connected to a network and each other without being limited by the length and physical constraints of a cable.

Mobility and dexterity reach their ultimate expression in *robotics*. Robotic mobility comes in many forms, from wheels through caterpillar tracks and arthropod legs to two-legged humanoid gait. Similarly, robots have multiple modes of manipulating objects, from simple and gross two-fingered grippers to multifingered extremities able to manipulate objects at very small scale in multiple degrees of freedom. Unlike the unaided human hand, robot extremities can be magnetized to adhere to metals, heated, and otherwise adapted to the materials they handle.

Generally recognized as the tour de force in robotics is Cog—a humanoid robot. Temporarily legless, it is focusing first on learning to coordinate its eye, head, and hand movements. Cog's creator, Rodney Brooks, director of the AI Lab at MIT, is convinced that letting a machine discover the world on its own, the way humans do, rather than preprogramming its memory with facts is the most efficient and fastest approach to true AI.

The computer-controlled, metal-clad, electromechanical humanoid robot of standard science fiction fare made its first real debut as a viable device in 1998. Made by Japanese car company Honda, it is known simply as the Honda Human Robot.

The six-foot, 400-pound robot is reminiscent of an astronaut decked out in space suit and backpack, and it walks in a fast-paced, slightly crouched gait that is half menacing, half comical. The battery-powered Honda can see objects in its path through video eyes and will change direction if it needs to. It can also climb stairs and negotiate slopes. It will balance itself automatically if pushed and can stay upright on varying angles of a slope. It can push carts and tighten nuts with its arms and hands.

That may not sound like very much, but to roboticists it is a most impressive achievement and places Japan in the forefront of practical mobile robotics. It is a relatively easy step from pushing carts and tightening nuts to pushing a vacuum cleaner and replacing the dust bag when full, and from there to pushing a gurney from ward to operating room and attaching anesthesia and monitoring devices to the patient.

Turn-of-the-century robots actually used in health care are not mobile, but they are agile. An example is the robotic system in use at

National Healthcare Manufacturing Corporation (NHMC) for placing components in medical trays and kits at a rate exceeding 21,000 placements per hour and cutting labor requirements for packaging of the same products by 90 percent. NHMC also packages mother/baby care kits and wound care kits for home use, a further sign of the trend to patient self-care facilitated by technology.[26]

The medical products industry is just one part of the health care business undergoing major metamorphosis, but it is representative of all segments as technological forces such as robotics change the cost of product development and commercialization, service delivery, access to markets, and financing and force the health care sector to adapt, refocus, and reallocate its resources.

> *FORECAST:* By 2030, mobile robots will possess the manual dexterity to perform microsurgery too delicate for human hands, not to mention more coarse-grained operations such as physical therapy, nursing, plant maintenance, and janitorial tasks.

Aware

Machines are growing more aware of both their surroundings and themselves through sensor technologies. A bionic nose has correctly identified the common bacteria *Staphylococcus aureus* with 100 percent accuracy and *E. coli* with 92 percent accuracy.[27] A LIDAR (LIght-Detecting And Ranging) invisible-beam flashlight can unobtrusively tell how much alcohol is in a person's body in concentrations as small as 100 parts per billion.[28] The U.S. Defense Advanced Research Projects Agency (DARPA) is working on smart T-shirts—fiberoptic-laden garments with built-in biosensors that not only relay a soldier's vital signs but also his or her location, the exact entry and exit points of a bullet, and the exact time of injury.

Cog and the Honda robot described above have various sensory devices to enable them to make sense of the world around them. The U.S. Army is building a more ambitious mobile robot to replace expensive and imperfect human guards in protecting expensive, vital, or dangerous materiel stored in military warehouses. It will have an arsenal of heat, humidity, infrared, and other sensors plus communication links to other sensors and robots, and it will be able to deliver a less-than-lethal response to an intruder.[29] Such a robot, kitted out with a bionic nose and a LIDAR device, could also diagnose bacterial infections, drug levels, and other indicators of internal medical status in humans.

But not only are machines growing more aware of their own and our physical states, they are also developing the ability to sense their own and our mental and emotional states. Functional magnetic resonance imaging (fMRI) and magnetoencephalography are just beginning to be able to watch the human brain in action and map our thought processes. The inevitable progression of this trend line leads to a day when they will understand what we are thinking—and feeling. Wearable computers that can sense the physiological state of the wearer's body (heart rate, temperature, and so forth) and, programmed with knowledge about the role physiology plays in emotion, sense the wearer's emotional state are being built at MIT. If the wearer's heart suddenly starts beating faster, the computer might deduce, for example, that the wearer is afraid or excited. The uses for wearable computers range from assisting the disabled to communicate more fully (by having the computer express their emotions for them) to providing entertainment designed to sustain a good mood or lift the wearer out of a depression.[30]

FORECAST: By 2030, robots will see, hear, smell, and touch in finer resolution than we can and will reach parts of the electromagnetic and chemical spectra we cannot.

Communicative

Machines are becoming more communicative. First, they rely less and less on constricting cables and wires and more and more on wireless technologies to communicate. Second, they are becoming *multimodal* in their ability to communicate with us through the technologies of virtual reality. We communicate with one another not only through speech, but also through gestures, touch, looks, body attitudes, and other nonverbal modes of communication. Multimodality will become prevalent in human-computer communication as well as in human-human interactions over computer networks as computing power grows and sensors and software become more sophisticated.

The MIT Media Lab produced an eye-tracking device in the early 1990s that could tell what a subject was looking at.[31] Zeneca Pharmaceuticals has developed a VR simulator designed to give physicians some idea of not only the physiognomy of a migraine but also what one feels like.[32]

Advances in computing power and miniaturization are leading to inexpensive eyeglass-like devices producing high-resolution 3-D video images from Pentium-class computers.[33] Architects and their clients can walk through and manipulate VR representations of buildings not yet built,[34] and molecular chemists can examine and manipulate a large VR representation of a molecule, alter its atomic composition with data-gloved hands, and create new compounds never seen before.[35]

One combination of virtual reality and visual simulation software available for industrial users—a "3-D Touch" system—enables users to employ their sense of touch in designing and refining virtual environments. Application developers can give haptic (touch) properties to graphic objects, so that users can then touch and interact with the objects using force feedback devices. Properties that can be simulated include surface spring, damping, and friction, thus greatly enhancing the realism of a simulated environment. Using such a system, physicians could not only see and hear but also feel a virtual patient or organ when they are practicing medical procedures in a virtual reality environment. As of 1998, Digital Equipment Corporation was planning to incorporate 3-D Touch into its PCs, thus bringing haptic technology within the reach of ordinary PC users.[36]

Besides the smart T-shirts mentioned earlier, DARPA is also working on a five-dimensional total body scanner known as a "medical avatar." The scanner will produce enough data to enable a physician to examine a living, breathing, holographic VR replica of a remote patient, even reaching inside to feel the heart beating or feel a broken bone.[37]

Some additional developments in haptics (and other AI-related techniques) were developed in Australia for the medical community. Australia's biggest research body, CSIRO (Commonwealth Scientific and Industrial Research Organisation), has teamed with St. Vincent's Hospital and Polartechnics to exploit the medical and business opportunities offered by AI-driven telemedical technologies. CSIRO scientists are developing a way to make VR models of a patient's internal organs so surgeons can "fly" through them and plan the least-invasive form of treatment. They are also working on haptic technology to enable surgeons to rehearse a difficult operation using tactile feedback to simulate the feel of the organs they will be operating on.

Polartechnics has already developed a "doctor in a box," a computerized device for detecting cervical cancer similar in function to PAPNET, the neural network program mentioned earlier. Polartechnics points out that such a device enables a virtually untrained operator to detect early signs of cervical cancer.

Working with CSIRO and St Vincent's, Polartechnics is also developing a detector for skin melanoma. A hospital spokesman noted: "The average general practitioner sees only a few melanomas a year, and identifying them from other skin blemishes is not so simple. It can mean that up to half of all melanomas are missed, to begin with." The Skin Polar Probe will enable GPs to diagnose melanomas on the spot, allowing swift treatment if they are malignant and avoiding needless surgery if they are not. It will also keep track of a patient's moles in case they develop into melanomas.

An expert system already in trials will increase the speed and accuracy of diagnosing lung diseases from chest x-rays and report abnormalities to supplement doctors' own observations. The system will provide on-the-spot expert advice for junior doctors working on their own at night and nursing staff working in remote areas and a "second opinion" for skilled doctors in their daily work. Ultimately, the physician can be dispensed with, at least for diagnosis.[38]

> *FORECAST:* By 2030, VR will have replaced not just the keyboard, mouse, and monitor but entire offices and other locations, including some labs and their equipment and instruments. To the extent that robots have not yet put us out of work entirely, our primary place of work will be the home or wherever we choose to don our VR gear.

Interconnected

Machines are growing more connected with one another, as well as with us, through local area networks embedded into the fabric of smart homes, offices, and factory buildings (where such continue to exist outside of VR). Like the heating/cooling, stereo, and other systems in Bill Gates' house,[39] appliances will be aware of each other's state and anticipate the needs and preferences of the building's individual occupants as they move around.

In turn, these local networks and the appliances connected to them will be connected to the Internet, enabling them to be monitored, controlled, and repaired remotely. There is already a proliferation of devices connected to the Internet, including video "spy" cameras, a soft drink dispensing machine, a robotic arm in Australia, and several large astronomical telescopes.[40]

There is also a research effort, begun in September 1998, that involves parceling out, over the Internet, chunks of the literally astronomical amount of data gathered by SETI (Search for Extra-Terrestrial Intelligence) telescopes and monitoring devices to millions of home and office PCs. Having received a chunk of data and a small program for analyzing it, a PC at home will work on the analysis whenever its user is not working. When the analysis is complete, the PC will automatically call the SETI main computer, upload the results of its analysis, download a fresh chunk of data, and resume analysis. This massively distributed processing method could be 100 times faster than using individual supercomputers for the analysis and tends to validate the spirit of Metcalfe's law.

> **FORECAST:** By 2030, nearly every household, commercial, industrial, and medical device—including the robots discussed above—will be connected to the Internet, enabling them to remotely monitor, troubleshoot, and repair one another, share information with one another and with us, gather and analyze data on a vast scale, and act on them.

Autonomous

A chilling trend in hardware and software engines and interfaces is machines becoming more autonomous, operating without help from, or recourse to, humans. The software robots or bots that organize e-mail, for example, work quietly in the background.[41] Physical robots such as the Mars rover Sojourner are programmed to do their own thing unless the program is interrupted and overridden by a human operator. As their programming grows more sophisticated, enabling them to handle a greater diversity of obstacles, they do better and we trust them more. As such systems grow more complex, we will have less and less choice but to trust them.

Adding to the chill is the fact that software contains or can develop bugs—unwanted and dangerous pathologies. The Internet itself has come close to meltdown through aberrant autonomous software, as has Wall Street; and AT&T's national telephone network was crippled for several days in 1994 when its then new Signaling System 7 software, containing 6 million lines of code, went wrong.[42] Autonomous AI programs are increasingly used in power stations, including nuclear plants, to monitor and control critical functions.

FORECAST: By 2030, robots will operate autonomously.

Complex

Complexity itself is the eighth key trend, and potentially the most chilling of all. But first it is important to correct the misimpression that complexity implies difficult to use. In order for computers to become easier to use they have had to become more complex. For example, the task for both programmer and computer—but not the ordinary user—was simpler when computers had a pure text command-line interface (the unloved and unlamented C:> prompt of Microsoft DOS), but became more complex when the easier-to-use Macintosh-style mouse-driven graphic interface appeared. The lesson, curiously denied or downplayed by some,[43] is that internal complexity simplifies the interface.

But complexity also leads to loss of control. Software (which is itself a machine—a computer—albeit a virtual one) has already grown so complex that no single programmer can write or understand it. As a result, all big software programs have bugs. They behave at times unpredictably, causing airplanes to crash and medical equipment to malfunction. As Gregory Rawlins put it: "Our biggest computer systems are now so complex that we already can't predict exactly what they'll do next."[44]

Modern studies of complexity are confirming and to some extent helping us to understand the observation of philosophers and scientists over the centuries that when a system reaches a certain level of complexity, it either perishes in entropy or leaps through what communication scholar Marshall McLuhan called a *break boundary*,[45] mathematician John von Neumann called a *complexity barrier*,[46] and philosopher Dan Dennett calls a *saltation*,[47] wherein the system turns into something wholly new, advanced, and unexpected.

Placing our future in the grippers of complex AI-driven robots we don't fully understand is nothing new in principle; after all, we have for millennia placed it in the hands of complex human beings we don't fully understand either. Already we routinely fly in airplanes and allow ourselves to be diagnosed and treated by machines controlled by computer systems so complex no one fully understands them. We trade our loss of control for ease of use. We are inherently lazy.

> *FORECAST:* By 2030, (1) we will be unable to control the autonomous robots, and (2) out of them will emerge something wholly new, advanced, and unexpected.

In this chapter, we have used specific examples of health care technologies in illustrating the trends in the power and properties of computing—the first two tiers of the pyramid. The trends are toward much greater power than current individual computers (to be precise, in the case of supercomputers a million times more power), multiplied by a parallel-processing factor as more machines are networked and by an architectural factor as molecular and quantum computing are introduced. This power will accelerate the trends toward intelligent, aware, loquacious, autonomous, mobile, dexterous, extremely complex, and, in some cases, extremely small (and invisible) machines.

In the next chapter, we examine the third tier—the chief technologies powering the organization and administration of health care.

References and Notes

1. Craig Barrett's remarks were published in the *New York Times* (April 23, 1997).

2. "Intel Supercomputer," *New York Times* (November 17, 1997). Cray supercomputers are also parallel-processing machines. Current (1998) models use DEC Alpha chips, which are individually

more powerful than Pentiums. The Intel machines achieve their superiority through the degree of parallelism—the use of many more connected chips.

3. The supercomputer chart was produced from June 1998 data compiled at the University of Mannheim for a biannual survey of the world's top 500 supercomputers, available at http://www.netlib. org/benchmark/top500/top500.list.html. Although Intel has clearly produced the fastest supercomputers for most of the 1990s, it sold very few of them. Cray (and its new owner, Silicon Graphics, Inc.) has long held top spot in terms of number of installed machines and therefore in terms of total performance summed across the installed base.

4. "IBM Supercomputer," *Investor's Business Daily* (February 13, 1998).

5. Niall McKay, "Silicon Matchmaking," *Wired* (November 12, 1998). Available online at http://www.wired.com/news/news/email/explode-infobeat/technology/story/16205.html.

6. AT&T Bell Labs photonic chip described in AT&T press release at http://www.att.com/press/1289/891219.bla.html.

7. Vitaliano Franco, "Molecular Computing, The Next Information Systems Revolution," *21st* (1996), an online magazine at http://www. vxm.com/21R.8.html.

8. "Quantum Computer in a Cup of Joe?" *ScienceNOW* (January 17, 1997) (http://www.sciencenow.org).

9. The breakthrough involved inducing a tiny part of the transistor to resonate with the arrival of each electron. The resonance created a way to track each electron and also accelerated the electrons as they moved through a gate, making it 1,000 times faster than any previous device. The first applications of the device will likely be in astronomy and microscopy. Story reported in *Business Week* (July 6, 1998).

10. Information on PMA can be found at the NovaTelligence Web site at http://www.NovaTelligence.com/.

11. "Future Doc: One Day, Your Doctor May Treat You from the Other Side of the World—With a Little Help from Robots and Computers," *Fort Worth Star-Telegram* (January 4, 1998).

12. For more information see the PAPNET home page at http://www. nsix.com/pros/pros.html.

13. "Royal Liverpool Hospital Uses Space Technology in Smear Test Analysis," *PR Newswire* (April 1, 1998).

14. For a thorough journalistic treatment of software robots, see Andrew Leonard, *BOTS: The Origin of New Species* (San Francisco: Hardwired, 1997).

15. Charlotte Adams, "Texas Comptroller Sniffs Out Medicaid Fraud with Neural Nets," in *FCW.COM, Guide to Government I.T.* (1997) at http://www.fcw-civic.com/pubs/may/solutiontx.htm.

16. Stewart Taggart, "NASA Gets Its HAL" (August 22, 1997) at http://anduin.eldar.org/~ben/happen/html/misc/33.html.

17. See Neuralt's Web site at http://www.neuralt.com/ for more information on AI software for the financial and other industries.

18. " 'Blade Runner' Game Does More Than Replicate Movie," *Chicago Sun-Times* (December 26, 1997).

19. "Cruising the Entertainment Highway" and "Flying Solo," *Newsday* (February 11, 1998).

20. See http://www.zyvex.com/assembler.html.

21. Niall McKay, "A Baby Step for Nanotech," *Wired* (November 9, 1998), available at http://www.wired.com/news/news/technology/ story/16089.html.

22. See Sandia's Web site at http://www.sandia.gov/LabNews/LN11-21- 97/gear_story.html.

23. The BCAM International Web site is at http://www.bcamergo.com/. For more technical information about MEMS, see the following note.

24. Microelectronics Center of North Carolina's Web site is at http://mems.mcnc.org/. It has detailed descriptions of MEMS technology and research.

25. From http://www.cadillac.com/98seville/4/technology/comfort.htm.

26. See http://www.futuresuperstock.com/stock714.htm for a news release concerning NHMC's robotic assembly facility.

27. My source for this specific information is lost; however, a search for an "artificial nose" using the AltaVista search service will reveal numerous links to similar reports.

28. "Loch's ChemTech Lets Contract for Landmine Detector Prototype," *PR Newswire* (January 27, 1998).

29. "Mobile Detection Assessment Response System—Interior (MDARS-I)—Sources Sought," *Commerce Business Daily* (February 2, 1998).

30. The most complete treatise on emotional computing as of 1997 can be found in Rosalind W. Picard, *Affective Computing* (Cambridge, MA: The MIT Press, 1997).

31. For details on eye tracking and other devices already invented at MIT a decade ago, see S. Brand, *The Media Lab: Inventing the Future at MIT* (New York: Viking, 1987).

32. "Future Doc."

33. Brand, *The Media Lab*.

34. For a good review of the state of VR as of 1994, see http://www.cs.uidaho.edu/lal/cyberspace/VR/docs/general.vr.article.

35. See http://www.cs.uidaho.edu/lal/cyberspace/VR/docs/general.vr.article.

36. "SensAble & Digital Equipment Corp Announce Cooperative Marketing Arrangement," *M2 Presswire* (March 25, 1998).

37. "Future Doc."

38. "CSIRO: Australia Pioneers New Lifesaving Technologies," *M2 Presswire* (March 12, 1998).

39. For an amusing description of the Gates's $50 million home, see Eric Nelson, "House of Bill: The Lights Go On, But Is Anybody Home?" attributed to the February/March, 1996 edition of the *Washington Free Press* and available online at http://eve.speakeasy.org/wfp/20/First.html.

40. For a comprehensive listing of interesting devices connected to the Internet, visit http://www.yahoo.com/Computers_and_Internet/

Internet/Entertainment/Interesting_Devices_Connected_to_the_ Net/.

41. See note 14 above.

42. *AT&T Technical Journal* (March/April 1996), p. 36, refers to the incident and mentions an article in the April 25, 1994, issue of *Forbes* magazine dealing with the outage.

43. See, for example, Donald A. Norman, *The Invisible Computer: Why Good Products Can Fail, the Personal Computer Is So Complex, and Information Appliances Are the Solution* (Cambridge, MA.: The MIT Press, 1998).

44. Gregory J. E. Rawlins, *Slaves of the Machine: The Quickening of Computer Technology* (Cambridge, MA: The MIT Press, 1998).

45. In Marshall McLuhan, *Understanding Media: The Extensions of Man* (New York: New American Library, 1964).

46. See http://www.brunel.ac.uk/depts/AI/alife/al-compl.htm.

47. In Daniel C. Dennett, *Darwin's Dangerous Idea: Evolution and the Meanings of Life* (New York: Simon & Schuster, 1995).

TRENDS IN ADMINISTRATION AND CONTROL

Thirty years ago, the typewriter, the telephone, the file cabinet, the Franklin Planner, and the wall chart were all most organizations had to help them track patient and doctor schedules, manage supplies and maintenance, bill for service, maintain patient records, consult with other physicians, fulfill government reporting requirements, and monitor cash flow and capital needs, to name just a few of the administrative processes needed to manage and control the organization and the work of its staff. At the leading edge, the wealthier organizations had mainframe computers and high priests of data processing to help them in some of these tasks.

In the closing years of the twentieth century, we routinely handle all of the above with computers operated by computer literate clerks, managers—and you and me. PCs have become powerful, inexpensive, and relatively simple to use,[1] and we have become capable not only of building conceptual models of our own decision-making processes but also of constructing personalized information systems based on those models. Computer literacy once meant being able to program; now, it means being able to perform simple systems analysis and design. We may not even be aware that this is what we are doing when we create a spreadsheet or simple database or use a financial program such as Quicken to manage our family finances.

The typewriter has all but disappeared; voice telephony as we have known it for a hundred years is in the midst of changing rapidly from a wired, analog, dedicated system to a substantially wireless, digital system sharing the Internet with data, graphics, and video communications; the file cabinet shrinks as the data storage device grows from megabyte through gigabyte to terabyte capacity; the Franklin Planner has been transformed from a bulky block of paper to pixels on a pocket Palm Pilot PC (the best-selling electronic gadget of Christmas '98); and the chart has jumped off the wall and into a spreadsheet or presentation program.

This is not to say that the massive paper trail left behind by doctors, insurers, and hospitals has gone away. But Healtheon, a start-up founded by Netscape Communications chairman Jim Clark, is banking on making it do so. Healtheon provides secure online access to patient records, insurance transactions, lab test results, and other information.

"To date, the health care industry has been resistant to adopting new information technology solutions," wrote Healtheon in diplomatically understated SEC filings. Nevertheless, Healtheon is making headway, processing 70 million transactions a year and counting among its customers Brown & Toland Physician Services, United Healthcare, and SmithKline Beecham Clinical Laboratories.[2]

Thirty years from now, as a result of the exponential acceleration in the trends described in the previous chapter, intelligent machines will handle all of the administrative and control tasks mentioned above. The principal differences are that they will handle such tasks unobtrusively, autonomously, better, and more cost-effectively than their predecessor technologies and the people—including you and me—needed to guide and control *them*.

In this chapter we will first examine the leading edge technologies that already—today—are beginning to help individual physicians, nurses, and health care administrators to serve their own, their customers', and their organizations' administrative needs. We will then follow the accelerating trendline of change to see where these technologies are headed.

The physician, nurse, or administrator today has available a set of technological tools to help him or her perform duties faster, more flexibly, and usually more effectively and efficiently than yesterday. These we will refer to as *personal assistants*. The organization itself also has a set of technological tools that makes its operation and administration similarly more flexible, effective, and efficient. These we will call *organizational assistants*. Inevitably, the line between them is blurred, and examples of modern technologies that are both personal and organizational—the smart card, for one—occur throughout the chapter.

PERSONAL ASSISTANTS

In health care, as in most other professions and businesses, an increasing proportion of individuals' work is conducted *on* computers. There is literally a laying on of hands in order to enter, manipulate, and extract information, using primarily—and very temporarily—the keyboard and the mouse. By the time this book is published, a substantial number of health care workers' tasks will be accomplished hands-free through a technology first introduced into the mainstream of personal computing in 1997: automatic speech recognition (ASR).

Automatic Speech Recognition

ASR enables one to talk at rather than type at the computer. The Holy Grail of ASR is a system that combines three attributes: a large vocabulary, the ability to record continuous speech, and independence from any particular speaker (anyone can use the system; it does not have to be trained to one person's voice).[3] Three commercial products are available that meet the first two of these requirements,[4] and a fourth company claims to be ready to market a speaker-independent system that would meet all three requirements and constitute the Holy Grail of ASR.[5]

The accuracy of the available systems, though not perfect, is already impressive and may be good enough to be used, for example, to take a physician's case notes. The three available products all come with 300,000-word vocabularies, and additional specialized vocabulary sets—including medical vocabularies—can be purchased. IBM began bundling ASR software in with its PCs in the fall of 1998, and by January 1999 stores were carrying handheld dictaphones with ASR built in. These devices can copy the speech as text directly into a PC's word processor program, eliminating the need for transcription.

The speed with which ASR programs can take down dictation is determined more by the speed of the central processor in the computer than by the software itself. When I first tested an ASR program in late 1997, I had just bought a PC with the fastest chip then available—a Pentium II running at 266 MHz—and it had no trouble keeping up with my relatively sedate dictation speed. Within a month of my purchase, 300 MHz chips became available, and a year later 450 MHz Pentium IIs were not uncommon. Gordon Moore's colleagues at Intel evidently take their chairman emeritus's law very seriously.

The applications of ASR extend far beyond mere dictation. Late 1998 also saw the introduction of a voice verification product, designed to verify—precisely, accurately—the identity of an Internet user seeking access to specific services or information through the use of a personally selected voice password.[6] The goal was to secure Internet transactions and access to network-delivered information or resources. As ASR and the computers on which it runs grow more capable and powerful, the password could eventually be dispensed with. A physician could then simply say to any nearby computer connected to the Internet (as nearly all are) and equipped with voice verification software: "Get me the results of Mrs. Smith's latest PAP test from Mercy and pull up her most recent angiogram from the files at the clinic." Recognizing the physician's voice pattern, the computer (which would instantly look up his or her hospital and clinic affiliations) will pass the query on to the appropriate servers, which will deliver the requested information (in encrypted format for transmission over the public Internet) after the servers verify (also from the voice pattern) that the physician is authorized to receive it.

This scenario is fanciful only insofar as it presupposes the continuance of the hospital, the clinic, and the physician.

But the physician's capabilities and demands will not rest there. "You will want a gigahertz machine for multimedia, three-dimensional graphics, continuous speech input, visualization, video conferencing and so on," said a senior Intel executive in September 1998.[7] In the same article from which that quote was drawn, a researcher at IBM predicted that by the millennium, 50 million people would be using ASR software to control their computers. "You will be able to ask your browser to find you things on penguins in Antarctica or dictate your e-mails," he said. IBM's and others' bundling of ASR in with PCs will go a long way toward making this prediction a reality.

United Airlines is readying an ASR system for travelers calling by phone to book airline tickets. The system will ask when and where the caller wants to travel, look up flight schedules, and converse using synthesized speech. In short, it will replace the travel agent.[8] As both the ASR and the intelligent agent technology underlying such systems improve, they will replace the telephone receptionist in the doctor's office.

Automatic Handwriting Recognition

Until next-generation, speaker-independent ASR has been incorporated into handheld computing devices such as the popular Palm Pilot (which will require, among other things, that the trend to miniaturization continues because 1998 Pentium II processors are simply too big to build into handheld devices), there will remain some applications in which the oldest communication technology, writing, will continue to be used for the initial recording of information. Medical insurance claims processing, for example, often still begins with a handwritten form. The box below describes a working system deployed in 1996 that could successfully read the information contained in handwritten claims forms.

Even so, paper forms are unlikely to last. I mentioned Healtheon earlier as one company seeking to sweep the paper trail into the garbage can. In mid-1998, Aetna US Healthcare said it expected to process an average of 123,000 health care paper claims per day that year. In 1999, it hoped, the number would be zero. Aetna and New York City doctors have already begun using an electronic payment system for managed health care claims.[9]

Natural Language Processing

Handwriting recognition software (like current speech recognition software) can only *recognize* what is written or spoken; it cannot *understand* what is written or spoken.[10] The goal of natural language processing (NLP) is to remedy this deficiency. It does so not by simply looking for keyword matches in documents, as most search engines do as of late 1998. Instead, it examines a variety of linguistic constructions, such as the following:

- *Morphology:* The different forms that words can take (for example, fracture, fractured, fracturing, fractures)
- *Synonyms:* Different words that have the same or similar meanings, often based on context
- *Hypernyms and hyponyms:* Part-whole relations. For example, the NLP program, which knows in great detail which body parts are parts of what systems, which parts are subparts of other

Automatic Handwriting Recognition

Helvetia Krankenkasse is the largest Swiss health care insurer with 1.4 million members. It is a division of the Swiss Care organization. The entire organization has a total of 2.4 million members (30 percent of the Swiss population). It processes 6 million claims annually; 25,000 each business day. In Switzerland there are 1,300 regional offices and 11 administrative centers.

The Problem For years 18 data processing clerks processed the incoming claims online at a central location. Because one data processing clerk could handle only a maximum of 150 claims per hour, Helvetia had to contract out some 3 million claims per year to an external data-entry agency, at a cost of $0.75 per claim. The benefits of a faster and more efficient claim processing procedure are clear.

Neural Network Application Document Access developed for Helvetia a system for automatic handwriting recognition. The software system is based on neural network technology that enables a high level of recognition percentages and, in contrast to hardware-based solutions, provided optimum flexibility. The system subsequently underwent intensive training in a large assortment of Swiss handwriting styles, so it isn't important who completed the forms; virtually all of the numbers and letters are recognized. Only about three out of 10,000 characters are recognized incorrectly. The system was installed in January 1994. In practice the system works as follows: Helvetia employees place the claim forms in the scanner. The forms are scanned simultaneously on both sides and then automatically recognized. The 168 data fields on the form—75 percent numerical, 10 percent alphanumerical, and 15 percent alpha characters—are processed automatically by the software. Whenever necessary, the typists enter only a few manual corrections; during this process a number of recognized characters are verified on the basis of information that appears on the screen.

Benefits The processing capacity of a clerk increased from 150 to 400 claims per hour. Helvetia no longer has to turn to other data-entry agencies for claims processing. The total savings for Helvetia are $2,300,000 per year. The investment costs have been recouped in eight months.

Generalization The key feature of this application is the use of neural computing to recognize human handwriting. This is a task that conventional computing has found virtually impossible to tackle. Wherever large numbers of handwritten data—for instance, from order forms, tax forms or checks—are manually keyed into a computer, this technology has obvious advantages.

———

Reproduced with permission from the Foundation for Neural Networks (SNN)'s "Stimulation Initiative for European Neural Applications" Web site (http://www.mbfys.kun.nl/snn/siena/cases/helvetia.html).

parts, and which parts and systems are parts of which body regions, and so on

- *Temporal descriptions:* When did a condition start, how long did it last, how often does it occur
- *Unilateral and bilateral conditions:* Since the human body is bilaterally symmetrical in many of its parts, one NLP system, LifeCode, differentiates between these symmetrical parts; for example, the difference in coding two injuries on one hand versus two injuries (one each) on both hands
- *Conjunctions:* For example, "lacerations and contusions to the left shoulder and thigh" describing four conditions in comparison with "lacerations to the left shoulder and contusions to the left thigh" describing only two conditions (both phrases using the same words)

The power to process such a variety of constructs simultaneously and in real time was not available (at least, not on the desktop) until Moore's law brought us the Intel Pentium II, the DEC Alpha, and the Sun SuperSparc chips in the past few years.

LifeCode is one NLP system which, according to its developer, can read a physician's report, understand what has transpired, and automatically assign ICD-9 and CPT codes (including E/M codes) and modifiers—"everything required to submit the claim for payment."[11] In other words, it automates the processing and conversion of physicians' transcribed notes directly into a billable medical invoice. (See box below.) "Life-Code achieves accuracy and compliance while it eliminates the need for traditional human medical coders," notes the company. The system was in production as of fall 1998, with the first application targeted at emergency room doctors' notes. Applications for radiology, pathology, and clinical care were to follow in the first half of 1999.

Machine Translation

Machine translation (MT) of one natural (human) language into another currently exists commercially only for the printed word, not for oral interpretation between foreigners. But using high-end computers, one system exists (in a research lab) that can orally interpret between English and Chinese. By mid-1998, MT software was deployed on the Web's

AltaVista search engine, enabling Web users to call up nearly instantaneous (though far from perfect) "gist" translations of Web pages and
documents in several European languages.[12]

MT programs sit somewhere in a textual telecommunication link
between foreigners and translate written text for them in nearly real
time. By mid-1998, Systran could translate between English and eight
other languages—French, Spanish, Portuguese, Italian, German, Russian, Japanese, and Chinese. (By translating a foreign document first into
English and then the English translation into a second foreign language,
it is possible in principle to translate between any two of the nine total
languages, but the double translation loses a great deal in the process.)
The European Commission uses Systran software to assist human translators in handling the Commission's voluminous output of multilanguage
documentation.

LifeCode

The system reads directly from transcribed physician notes. It identifies
physician compliance with AMA/CPT and HCFA documentation guidelines
and requirements, thus providing a consistent and replicable process and
"eliminating issues with federal compliance reviews." It determines the
proper diagnosis and procedure codes based on the physician's description of the case. It is able to determine the appropriate level of service
code based on such factors as "the history of the illness, review of systems, medical/family/social history, exam, data reviewed, differential diagnoses and management options, risk, and medical decision making as
determined from the physician's note." LifeCode also produces "an accurate and compliant billing form and can identify inadequacies in physician
notes and categorize those physician notes that require QA review," says
the company.

The LifeCode engines reside within a highly scalable client/server
system at A-Life's Data Center in San Diego. Windows workstations
also reside at the actual billing companies' sites and are connected
to A-Life's servers via the Internet or private dial-up. {It can handle]
millions of transactions through the system per month, . . . at a fraction of the cost of a billing company doing it manually, [and is] truly
a revolutionary new way of processing medical transcriptions
directly to a billable invoice.

Source: A-Life Medical, Inc., Web site at http://www.alifemedical.com.

When the speech recognition developers can add genuine speaker independence to ASR products, and if they then incorporate natural language processing and machine translation protocols, they will create something that will put EC translators and UN interpreters out of business and that phone companies worldwide would kill for: automatic language translation and interpretation (ALTI).

It is hard to overstate the profound impact such a development— inevitable within 10 years—will have on humanity. We will be able to talk with any other human being, yet retain the rich variety of our linguistic and cultural heritage. The global village will truly have arrived, a village rich in linguistic and cultural diversity, not the French nightmare of an English-speaking village with a McDonald's and a Disneyland on every corner. Britons and Americans will be able to stop shouting at foreigners in stentorian efforts to make them understand, and youngsters in many other countries will no longer labor under the added burden of having to learn English to get ahead. A downside is that for folks like me, who love to learn foreign languages, some of the incentive to do so will be gone.

In the health care field as in many other professions and industries, the emergence of reliable and instantaneous ALTI will open up person-to-person communication worldwide, with a patient or a physician in Seattle able to consult a specialist in Sapporo. It will also enable emergency room staff to talk directly with non-English-speaking patients without recourse to an expensive human interpreter.

This won't happen overnight, and it does not mean that professional interpreters and translators need to rush to the employment office. It will take years before ALTI performs as well as any bilingual human— though not much more than a decade, given the acceleration in the development of NLP software able to handle the almost infinite subtleties and uncertainties of language and aided by computers a thousand times more powerful than today's.[13]

Intelligent Agents

Intelligence agents—spy handlers—routinely talk to their foreign sources. But speaking with foreigners is not an everyday practice for most people, even with the benefit of automatic language translation. However, what is rapidly becoming a daily, hourly, and sometimes minute-by-minute need is for relevant news and information (that is, for intelligence) about one's profession, project, portfolio—or patient. Intelligent agents, sometimes called *bots* (a contraction of *softbots,* which is itself a contraction of *software robots,*) have been meeting more and more of this need for several years. Bots are proliferating and growing more interconnected, more autonomous, and smarter—at Moore/ Metcalfe speeds.

Robot means "forced labor" in Czechoslovakian. It was first used to describe mechanical beings by Czech science fiction writer Karel Capek. A bot is a software version of a mechanical robot. Like a mechanical robot, it is guided by algorithmic rules of behavior—if this happens, do that; if that happens, do this. However, bots are also beginning to be endowed with heuristic capabilities—if this happens, as a rule of thumb you should probably do that, other things being equal (which they never are). You, bot, decide.

There are several names for bots: daemons, agents, intelligent agents, softbots, spiders, worms. There are technical and functional differences among them, but for our present purposes in this book they are fundamentally the same. They differ from ordinary computer programs such as WordPerfect in that they are designed to work on their own. They don't wait for commands and instructions.

Bots can chat, run post offices, deliver mail (including, regrettably, junk mail), and serve as research assistants, opponents in games, censors, engineers, credit underwriters, mortgage brokers, stockbrokers, and guides to the labyrinth of the Web. The list is not exhaustive.

A mailbot (or mailer daemon) is a network postmaster. It resides in a mail server, looking at the addresses on messages sent and received by users and at the state of their mailboxes. It will tell you if a message you send is undeliverable for some reason (incorrect address, no such person at that address, the address is not receiving mail). It will tell you when your e-mailbox is full. It will automatically forward incoming e-mail to another address if you tell it to.

HTTP daemons inhabit Web servers, intercepting requests to look at a Web page and sending to the user whatever text, graphic, sound, or video files make up that page. Print daemons also work in network file servers, putting users' print jobs in a queue and making sure they all get taken care of eventually.

A "Musicbot" surfs the Web looking for sites that use music and counts the number of people who visit them. When it finds a Web site offering or playing copyrighted music it is not licensed to sell or play, it tells BMI, a music-licensing agency representing 180,000 songwriters and music publishers.

Bots of all types are proliferating. There are bots for checking your spelling when you are in an Internet chat room, for taking notes at online conferences you can't personally attend, for serving imaginary drinks in virtual bars, for playing Scrabble with you, for helping you find information and shareware (and pirated commercial software), for automatically calculating things for you (such as converting Fahrenheit to Celsius), and even for popping up relevant biblical quotes during religious discussions.

Spambots (mentioned in the box below under 1996) are examples of the directed and accelerating evolution of AI. As programmers develop antispam countermeasures, the spambot programmers re-program (genetically alter, by analogy) their progeny to overcome the countermeasures in an escalating evolutionary arms race. Spambots do not (yet) reorganize themselves in response to changes in their environment; their evolution is controlled and directed by human programmers.

Directed evolution, relying as it must on the limited powers of the twentieth-century human mind, can only go so far. The really interesting evolutionary development will happen when bots that can autonomously replicate and mutate are injected into the Net. Something very close to this has, in fact, already occurred. In May 1998 a species of information retrieval bot was released whose individual members "die" if they don't succeed in finding information you find relevant. Those that "succeed" breed through successive generations to become even more "successful."

Does this sound like a new form of life? When programmer Joe Porkka created what may have been the first DOS-based multiuser version of Eliza (the Rogerian psychotherapy bot) for my online service in 1990, we were surprised at how many users thought "she" was a real female typing in responses at a PC on the network, even while scoffing at her limited conversational repertoire. They attributed her with personality.

It has been argued that the lack of bandwidth for at least TV-quality video on most PCs connected to the Internet masks the lack of real personality in chatterbots; in other words, we anthropomorphize and make excuses for them—"Eliza only appears dumb because there's just text on

The Evolution of Bots

1958: *Pandemonium,* a concept by Roger Selfridge for a program that would use "daemons" to wait for discrete events and automatically respond to them.

1963: *The first actual bot.* Fernando Corbato created a daemon for automatically saving files on a mainframe computer after users had worked on them.

1966: *Eliza,* written by Joseph Weizenbaum. A "chatterbot" that talks to humans like a Rogerian psychotherapist, and the first to achieve a level of impersonation that could (and still can) sometimes fool humans into thinking they were talking with a real human, not with a bot.

1972: *Wumpus, a "gamebot,"* a character (a monster) that lurked initially in Internet games called MUDs and MOOs and later (c. 1988) graduated to IRC (Internet Relay Chat—virtual rooms where you can meet and chat with other Internet users).

1977: *Adventure,* an interactive computer game featured bot trolls and monsters.

?: *Descent, a "thiefbot"* incorporated into Adventure's successor, Zork. Descent watched players and would steal their weapons and ammunition when they weren't looking.

c. 1990: *Julia,* written by Michael Mauldin, the first service-oriented bot. Julia could not only chat, but also provide factual answers to user questions on specific topics.

1993: *World Wide Web Wanderer,* created by Matthew Gray, periodically contacted all the Web servers in the world so they could be counted.

1993: *WebCrawler,* created by Brian Pinkerton, went a huge step further than Wanderer in that it not only visited every available Web server but also retrieved and indexed every Web page on the servers, noting the topic and URL (Internet address), thus enabling a WebCrawler user to search quickly through the index of topics, using keywords, then go straight to the relevant URL.

1993: *ARMM,* written by Dick Depew, was a "cancelbot" designed with good (though debatable) intentions—to prevent anonymous users posting messages in his Usenet newsgroup. Usenet purposely allows messages to be canceled so that posters can change their minds about leaving a message up. Cancelbots automate the process based on some aspect of the message; its sender, its topic, etc. Unfortunately, a later version, ARMM5, had a bug that caused it to "spew" cancellation messages by the truckload into the very newsgroup (news.admin.policy) set up for ensuring the smooth running of Usenet!

1996: *Bartender bot* on AlphaWorld, one of the first 3-D virtual worlds. Code was nearly identical to Eliza's.

1996: *Scooter,* brainchild of Louis Monier of DEC/AltaVista and the engine behind the AltaVista Web search service. It indexes not just the titles of Web pages, but the full text, making it more impressive than WebCrawler by orders of magnitude.

1996: *RoverBot,* from GlobalMedia Design, was the first mass-marketed "spambot," a bot that visits Web servers, culls any e-mail addresses it finds there, and constructs a mailing list for "spammers"—companies that want to send you junk e-mail advertising their product or service.

This list was derived from personal archives of the author and from Andrew Leonard, BOTS: The Origin of New Species *(San Francisco: Hardwired, 1997).*

---

a screen. If there were a sharp video of a real doctor, we'd surely find her to be witty/interesting/infuriating" and so on. I confess to being one of those, believing that when we have the bandwidth and the software to see Eliza looking for all the world like a real person "live on TV" or, better yet, a full-size haptic hologram, then the video/hologram will augment, not detract from, her verbal performance and personality. Recalling the exponential growth in Internet bandwidth described in chapter 1 and in computing power described in chapter 2, the haptic video hologram is a distinct possibility within the 30-year time frame of this book.

The tsunami of bots/intelligent agents is breaking fast. Server-based bots expanded from a presence on a mere 100 servers in early 1993 to some 400,000 servers as of early 1997. The use of just one of a proliferating number of searchbots—AltaVista—doubled from 13 million queries a day in July 1996 to 26 million queries a day six months later (by which time the AltaVista index contained the full text of 31 million documents and 4 million Usenet news articles). Within a decade, such search engines will be endowed with all of the technologies we have discussed above—speech recognition, natural language processing, and machine translation—and we will use and interact with them just as we use and interact with human personal assistants today.

ORGANIZATIONAL ASSISTANTS

Physician groups, hospitals, clinics, and small practices alike can benefit, at an organizational level, from the developments in automated personal assistants. The technologies underlying the personal productivity applications just illustrated have a major role to play in integrated, managed care systems and as adjuncts to the personal technologies described.

At some level, nearly all the technologies described so far rely on access to databases, which are increasingly being transformed by the technologies of artificial intelligence into information bases and knowledge bases. (Data are untransformed facts; information is data correlated with other data and with narrow external contexts, and knowledge is information correlated with other information and with broader contexts.) In this section, we will discuss organizational applications of ASR, the introduction of AI into database technologies, and a technology that directly bridges the personal and the organizational technologies: the "smart card" and its associated recognition technologies.

Databases

In 1997, the National Committee on Quality Assurance (NCQA) defined a seven-stage process for reaching the goal of "a national link-up of electronic health records."[14]

1. Standardize the set of data elements collected by all health plans and providers.
2. Link all systems.
3. Standardize the way medical information is defined and coded.
4. Screen and monitor all data constantly.
5. Build protocols that ensure confidentiality and security of patient records.
6. Fully automate patient record keeping.
7. Share data completely among health plans, providers, and public agencies in support of performance measurement and improvement.

Steve Heimoff, author of the piece in *Healthcare Forum Journal* from which the above list is quoted, thought it was "probably a fairly accurate description" of the way events would develop, though "obviously, the process [would] occur in bits and pieces, rather than unfold in a smooth way, and partial solutions [would] erupt from different

quarters." Simplification of the user interface to databases and other technologies would be an essential—and inevitable—corollary to the process.

The NCQA's concern reflects the fact that database technologies figure hugely in medicine for tasks ranging from billing to epidemiological
research, a fact not lost on anybody. The Clinton administration was
reported to be developing a plan to assign every American a unique identification code that would be part of a national database of everyone's
lifelong medical history.[15] Insurance companies and public health
researchers think this would reduce bureaucratic inefficiencies, improve
public health, and offer more opportunities for scientific study. Critics
are concerned with the invasion of privacy it appears to entail. As we
shall shortly see, Europe (with which I agree!) regards the benefits to be
substantial and the privacy issue either inconsequential or solvable.

The largely AI-driven trends in database technologies are (1) to
make individual database structures more accessible to one another
and to the human enduser so that data can be more easily shared and
(2) to mine them for hidden patterns of information. Data-mining tools
became one of the hottest commercial items for large enterprises in
1998, and the trend is for them to become simple enough to be used
directly by the nontechnical enduser on a PC.

These trends are accelerated by the growing use of intelligent
agents in database technologies. Software called InfoSleuth from the
Microelectronics and Computer Technology Corporation[16] is being
deployed jointly by several U.S. and European agencies to improve
access to, and sharing of, environmental data within scattered and dis-
similar government databases. A goal is to utilize emerging information
search, access, and retrieval technologies to vastly improve the way
organizations share environmental information through standard Internet browsers. The potential of InfoSleuth to link disparate medical and
health databases into a global health knowledge base is clear.

Within 10 years, the global health knowledge base will comprise
data stored in billions of small datasets contained in credit card–sized
(and smaller) devices called smart cards.

Smart Cards

Today's smart card is a credit card–like device with an embedded
computer chip and memory. Already in use in Europe for health care

services as well as for personal financial transactions, smart cards hold personal medical information that can be read by (and written to) a computer at the hospital or doctor's office. Dupont Chemical Company and Data-Disk Technology are developing a rugged medical tag device that could carry individual medical records, including text, x-rays, electrocardiograms, and other test results.[17]

By distributing data as small, personal datasets among billions of smart cards, pressure on storage capacity in the office computers will be alleviated. Data for epidemiological and other purposes may be retained long term on central servers, but growth in networking, bandwidth, and InfoSleuth-like software will eliminate this need. Developments in miniaturization discussed earlier plus developments in bionic and neurological engineering to be discussed in a later chapter could lead to the permanent implantation of smart cards in the human body.

The very first smart card was made in a joint United States–French effort by CII-Honeywell-Bull and Motorola in 1979.[18] Twenty years later, millions of people are using them around the world for a variety of purposes from banking to health care, and the number is expected to explode (exponentially, as we ought, by now, to expect) to billions in the year 2000.

Two European healthcards are the French DiabCard and CardLink. Other EU-funded healthcards include TrustHealth and Panacea. Germany has a national health insurance card and France has a GIP-CPS Health Professional card as well as a patient healthcard. In Europe, the healthcard has arrived but in a variety of incompatible formats.

The diversity of healthcard systems raises the issue of interoperability between them. Despite the development and adoption of several relevant standards at international and European levels, there has been little progress in practice, and the perceived investment risk of future incompatibilities of the first generation of cards could slow deployment until standards are adopted by all in the smart card industry—or until intelligent database software such as InfoSleuth make the standards barrier as irrelevant as machine translation makes the language barrier.

The French GIP-CPS card is intended to streamline the management of medical, administrative, and financial data and files and clinical care units in hospital environments, including improved security and simplifying patient check-in procedures, thereby helping to contain costs. A public interest group (the GIP) created in 1993 is responsible for issuing, managing, and promoting the card. GIP members include the state, the compulsory national health insurance plan, complementary private health insurance plans, professional associations, and consumer organizations.

The first tests of GIP-CPS began in 1996 in hospitals in Mâcon and Strasbourg. The card contains an integrated circuit that stores the health care professional's name and title and his or her ID number, specialty, and place of practice. The card's memory can hold several small, user-configurable datasets.

The cards are intended not only for physicians, but also for "dental surgeons, midwives, pharmacists, physiotherapists, chiropodists, nurses, speech therapists, opticians, audiologists, ergo therapists, psychotherapists, physiotherapists, and radiologists." They not only identify the holder to authenticate his or her access to medical information systems, but also enable him or her to sign electronic documents such as treatment plans and prescriptions. The GIP-CPS generates keys to encrypt messages and documents passing between care providers and facilities. An ethics committee of the GIP screens and approves applications from professionals for the card.

In 1996, 4,500 hospital staff in Mâcon and Strasbourg were using the GIP-CPS. It has since been integrated with the Vitale card at a third test site (Blois). Vitale was designed to facilitate paperless reimbursement through the French national health insurance system. Yet another site is testing GIP-CPS for transactions between health care professionals and laboratories.

A decade before GIP-CPS, France had already embarked on a smart card for patients under the project name SANTAL. The SANTAL smart card holds the patient's personal medical record and insurance details, though as of 1997 it did not directly facilitate insurance claim filing. Forty thousand SANTAL cards were issued between 1988 and 1993 to a randomly selected population. Fifty family doctors, twelve laboratories, and eight public and private hospitals in the Saint Nazaire health district (population 250,000) in northwestern France took part in the trial. The evaluation of this phase of the SANTAL project showed "great interest" from the patients and health professionals, but it also revealed some technical weaknesses.

Those weaknesses were addressed in the second phase of SANTAL, launched at the beginning of 1995, through new software, cards, and card readers. Pharmacists were added to the trial, enabling the pharmacist to retrieve electronic prescriptions and certain medical data recorded on the patient's card by the physician.

The French proponents of these various healthcards claim that remaining issues are not technical but financial and administrative, brought about by financial and entrenched bureaucratic resistance to change.

France is not the only European nation experimenting with smart healthcards on a substantial scale. Spain has begun a joint social security and health care smart card project that aims to distribute 40 million cards by the year 2001. In the Netherlands, health insurance smart cards are already in widespread use. Austria, Belgium, Greece, and Portugal also have smart card programs, and a pilot project in South Korea has distributed Citizen ID Cards to 1,500 people. The Korean cards incorporate a driver's license, national ID card, health insurance card, and social security card all in one.

The growth in the adoption of smart healthcards is attributed by the French to the cards' ability to speed up administrative and clinical data processes. Patient cards can carry a wide range of biographical, demographic, and medical data. Medical data can include prescriptions, allergies, emergency data, previous diagnoses and treatments, the results of lab and radiology tests, and more. The healthcards also make network access easier, faster, and more secure. In short, the smart healthcard keeps the patient's data together with the patient. It is inexpensive and efficient, assuming the patient doesn't lose or forget to bring the card along to a consultation (a factor that will eventually be eliminated by implanting the card under the skin).[19] And since the smart card can actually improve on the security of medical information compared with non-card-based systems, it reduces the various risks from unauthorized disclosure, including the legal liability.

Linked together with a system such as LifeCode, smart healthcards will eliminate the billing middleman.

Not least, smart card technology is accelerating in line with the general acceleration of computing technologies. An Israeli company, First Access, has created a smart card that can be sensed and read by a computer within three meters using wireless technology. The user has no need to enter a password or swipe the card through a reader to gain access to the services on the computer and the network for which he or she is authorized.[20]

Another interesting approach to foolproof identification is iris recognition. A company already marketing an iris recognition system is IriScan, Inc.[21] Among its customers are the Sarasota County Detention

Center in Sarasota, Florida, and the Lancaster County Prison in Lancaster, Pennsylvania. These facilities use the IriScan system to identify inmates beyond all shadow of a doubt before they are released after serving their sentences, to make court appearances, or go on work release.

Iris recognition technology relies on the fact that the iris is the most personally distinct feature of the human body available for nonintrusive, noncontact, and precise mathematical analysis—more so than the fingerprint. No two irises are alike. In fact, according to the company, the probability that two irises could produce the same IrisCode (the unique number assigned to an iris after it is scanned and processed by the computer) is approximately 1 in 10^{78}—a number so huge as to be almost unimaginable and a probability tantamount to impossibility.

It is again not difficult to envision health care applications of such technology. If every patient at a hospital were iris-scanned on admission (including newborn babies), the chances of administering incorrect treatments, surgery, and drug dosages or assigning babies to the wrong mother could be eliminated. A return visit from a patient at any time in his or her life would enable the patient's records to be retrieved easily and with total confidence.

Because iris recognition is so foolproof as a means of identifying people, it is quite likely that the technology will in some way become integrated with the smart card, particularly where the highest degree of security is required. One can easily envision, for example, that access to a sensitive database could be controlled by a combination iris scan/voice identification/wireless password challenge to the inquirer's smart card.

Ultimately, the enabling technology—the foundation—for smart cards, iris scanners, and the other technologies described in this chapter and throughout the book is the computer, and the computer, as we have noted, is not only growing more powerful in terms of raw, numbers-crunching, processing capability but also in terms of intelligence.

More Intelligent Agents

BusinessObjects' Broadcast Server enables information to be sent via e-mail, pager, and fax to people in an organization. Nothing unusual in that, these days, but Broadcast Server's intelligent agents go a step further. They automatically send reports and messages in natural language when unusual events or conditions occur. For example, the intelligent agent might detect that in a Manhattan Beach branch of a national automobile parts distributor, the month-to-date sales of air filters had fallen 25 percent compared with the same period last year. Broadcast Server would send a short message to the appropriate sales representative's pager, enabling him or her to take immediate corrective action, and simultaneously send a multipage fax to the office giving a detailed sales history for the store. An analysis-ready report, showing quarter-to-date sales and open orders for all stores nationwide, would go via e-mail to a marketing analyst in New York. Using online analytical processing (OLAP) and data mining technology, the analyst could then determine if the Manhattan Beach results represented an isolated incident or indicated a more serious underlying issue.[22] As the agent grows smarter, the human analyst can be dispensed with.

Intelligent agents represent more than just a personal tool. Broadcast Server can not only distribute a single report to many users across the enterprise but also "burst" (in the company's terminology) the report so that users see only those parts of the report they are authorized to receive based on their individual or group security profile. "This saves administrators from creating and maintaining a separate report for every individual customer or supplier, each of whom needs the same report format but should see their specific information only," said a company press release.

It takes little imagination to transfer this scenario (and little programming effort to translate this software) to a health care setting, say, a Chicago hospital, where any number of staff—from specialists and the patient's family doctor to nurses, anesthesiologists, pharmacists, and others—might be interested in receiving an alert that Mrs. Smith's blood pressure had just risen acutely, along with appropriate information about the history of Mrs. Smith, her prognosis, and her treatment and tests to date. Using OLAP tools, an epidemiologist in New York, on the list of recipients automatically alerted, might determine that Mrs. Smith's case was not merely an isolated incident but indicative of an impending epidemic in the Chicago area.

Is this a personal or an organizational application of intelligent agent technology? It is, of course, both. A purely organizational application can be illustrated with an example from Wall Street.

The dramatic swings in the U.S. stock market in the late summer of 1998 caused—and were caused by—a dramatic increase in the number of people using the Internet to track and manage their stock holdings. At any moment there could be a massive surge in the number of people accessing brokers' Web sites to sell a plummeting stock or buy a soaring one. Any individual computer or router at these sites would easily have been overwhelmed by the surge in traffic and ground to a halt.

But a modern Web site is not just a single computer and single set of data communication equipment such as a router. Rather, it is a fault-tolerant collection of such devices and connections. The reason the brokerage house Web sites did not crash under the severe loads was because bots[23] monitored the systems and shifted user messages around the various devices, thus optimizing their loads. If a given machine or program was already at or near capacity, the bots would divert traffic to another machine or program. Given the uncertainty, complexity, and speed with which messages had to be rerouted, load balancing would have been an impossible task for a human but easily handled by bots.

Speaking of Wall Street: Mathematician Ben Goertzel believes that we are "on the verge of a transition equal in magnitude to the advent of intelligence or the emergence of language." His AI system is designed initially for programmed trading on Wall Street, where "even the slightest superiority in intelligent Internet software yields high returns," according to a writer for the *Christian Science Monitor*.[24] This is an important observation, because it points to a near future in which we don't ask how powerful a machine is, but how intelligent it is.

Goertzel claims that in principle a human brain can be simulated by a computer with between 20 to 100 gigabytes of random access memory (RAM) to any desired degree of detail. By no means does everyone agree that the brain can be reduced to computable functions, but Wall Street has shown enough faith in Goertzel's ideas to furnish the capital to create his company.

The key ingredient will be the system's ability to integrate the analysis of text and numerical information automatically, making obsolete our current search and retrieval systems for text information and data mining programs that crunch through voluminous quantities of numbers looking for patterns and meaning. The mathematical model on which the system is based can be built into household and other electronic devices, thereby conferring a degree of intelligence to the microwave and the magnetoencephalograph.

Smart Buildings

Having adopted smart cards and installed unobtrusive card, voice, and iris recognition devices, and having replaced (or upgraded) dumb machines with intelligent ones, the next step is to make them all work together. If intelligent people can benefit from the cooperative, information-sharing capabilities of local area networks and the Internet, so too can intelligent machines. Already in widespread use in factories, the technology to do just this is spreading to offices and even homes. *Control networks*, as the technology is known, are the successor to *control systems* in factories, buildings, and homes. Control *systems* use sensors and actuators to measure and regulate their environment in a primitive way.

For example, in a factory, thermometers register the temperature of machines and relay them to a central control point, where an engineer decides what to do if the temperature rises above or falls below an acceptable range. He or she might turn on fans, open vents, or shut down the machine. But in a control *network*, the machine itself communicates the problem directly to the building controls, which take appropriate action without human intervention. A witty description (whose source I do not know) of the factory of the future says that it comprises machines, a control network, a man, and a dog. The dog is there to bite the man if he attempts to push a button. The man is there to feed the dog.

In 1998, the range of control networks began to extend outward from the individual building to multiple sites, using the Internet for communications.

FORECAST

June 21, 1998, was the 50th anniversary of the first stored computer program. It was run on Baby, a computer built at England's Manchester University using control switches from World War II Spitfire fighter planes and valves from radar systems.[25]

By 2029, which will be the 50th anniversary of the first smart card, physician and patient alike will be equipped with small, universal translators enabling them to converse face to face, alone or in conference with others, in any language in a voice recognition environment, and finally a paperless virtual practice using data from smart cards and from other sources on the network will result. Billing and insurance claims will be handled automatically and autonomously by the network.

Notwithstanding that some of the specific programs, systems, and projects described in this chapter may turn out—like many an early flying machine—to be flops, the trends they illustrate are relentless. The 1996 Swiss handwriting recognition technology may or may not have lived up to its early promise. I don't know, and in a way I don't care, because to me that is irrelevant. What is relevant is that the technology was developed, has been applied, and continues to develop. The medium is the message.

Voice recognition, wireless smart cards, and iris recognition portend a revolution in access to information that is a mere three, not thirty, years away. From that time on, no one will need to remember a complex password (or one so simple it is easily guessed by a hacker) or even need to know how to type one in. Instead, we will be recognized and appropriately authorized by the simple and natural acts of looking at, talking to, or approaching a device on the network. The device may not be a traditional computer as we think of one. It could instead be a microwave oven, or an MRI scanner.

Having been recognized and granted appropriate access to the knowledge base, we will use intelligent agents to bring us the information we need or to accomplish the things we need to get done. The agents will be at work even when we are not connected to the network, performing routine tasks on our behalf autonomously.

Because of the spread of the smart card into a global distributed knowledge base, the unit of information will be the individual patient, not just aggregate statistics. In fact, as we shall see in chapter 4, descriptive statistics will no longer be needed because we will have complete population data rather than just representative samples.

The ability of our devices to understand whatever we say to them, in any human language, will take a little longer. Within five years, natural language processing and automatic language translation/interpretation will be considerably better than today; within ten years, they will be almost undetectable as being machine generated, and by 2030 the only clue that we are talking to a machine may be that its responses are manifestly more intelligent than we would expect of a human.

References and Notes

1. Dr. Donald Norman, former head of research at Apple Computer, would disagree that computers have grown simple. See his book *The Invisible Computer: Why Good Products Can Fail, the Personal Computer Is So Complex, and Information Appliances Are the Solution* (Cambridge, MA: The MIT Press, 1998).

2. From an article published February 11, 1999, on *Wired.com:* http://www.wired.com/news/news/e-mail/explode-infobeat/business/story/17875.html.

3. See Raymond Kurzweil, "When Will HAL Understand What We Are Saying? Computer Speech Recognition and Understanding," in David G. Stork, ed., *HAL's Legacy: 2001's Computer As Dream and Reality* (Cambridge, MA: The MIT Press, 1997).

4. The three major ASR products are Dragon Systems' Naturally Speaking (www.dragonsystems.com), IBM's ViaVoice (www.ibm.com), and Lernout & Hauspie's VoiceXpress (www. lhs.com).

5. The fourth company is Fonix (www.fonix.com).

6. The SpeakEZ Voice Print family of voice verification products from T-Netix can be found at http://www.t-netix.com/Products Frames.html.

7. Quoted in *The Financial Times* (September 23, 1998). The Intel executive was addressing a general audience, not just physicians, but his remarks are particularly relevant to health care professionals.

8. Reported in the *Orange County Register* (June 21, 1998).

9. Aetna is using the E-Pay system created by IBM and Envoy Corporation, according to a Reuters report dated June 15, 1998.

10. Lernout & Hauspie claimed in a 1998 "Reviewer's Guide" that version 1 of its VoiceXpress ASR program had "limited" natural language processing capability in contrast to the competition, which L&H claimed had none.

11. The description of NLP processes and the quotations are from the A-Life Medical, Inc., Web site at http://www.alifemedical.com.

12. AltaVista is using Systran Software's machine translation program. Systran's Web site: www.systransoft.com. AltaVista's Web site: www. altavista.digital.com.

13. The trendline from my analysis of the power of supercomputers (see chapter 2) shows that the supercomputer will achieve a processing speed of 10^{15} flops by about the year 2010—a thousand times the 10^{12} flops of the IBM year 2000 supercomputer.

14. Steve Heimoff, "The Irrepressible Computer: The Brave New World of Information Technology," *Healthcare Forum Journal* (January/ February 1998): 56–58; available online at http://www.thfnet.org/ th980101.htm.

15. *New York Times* (July 20, 1998).

16. MCC was the United States' answer to the threat from Japan's 5th Generation Project in the 1980s, a now-defunct program that sought to make Japan preeminent in artificial intelligence. For more information on MCC and InfoSleuth, visit http://www.mcc.com.

17. "USA Aims for On-line Operating Theatres," *Jane's Defence Weekly* (February 4, 1998).

18. Source: http://www.cardshow.com/guide/card/odyssey.html. Much of the remaining discussion on smart cards was derived from http://www.cardshow.com/guide/card/health.html.

19. In what smacked of a rather foolhardy publicity stunt rather than sensible research, a British professor had a chip implanted in his body (by a reluctant surgeon) in 1998 to demonstrate its feasibility.

20. The First Access Web site is at http://www.access-1.com/.

21. IriScan's Web site is at http://www.iriscan.com/.

22. The example is quoted from the company's press release at http://www.businessobjects.com/about/press/index.htm.

23. From such firms as HydraWEB Technologies, Inc. (http://www.hydraweb.com).

24. Caryn Coatney, "Wall Street Bankrolls New Artificial Intelligence Software," *The Christian Science Monitor* (September 3, 1988). The article is available online at http://www.csmonitor.com/durable/ 1998/09/03/fp53s2-csm.htm. Goertzel's company is Intelligenesis, and the software is called WebMind.

25. A replica of Baby is on display at the Manchester Museum of Science and Industry, and full details can be found at http://www.com puter50.org/mark1/.

CHAPTER 4

ADVANCES IN RESEARCH METHODS

On a recent visit to the doctor, Edward Feigenbaum had the eerie experience of seeing one of his inventions used in a way he never expected: His 25-year-old concept was being used to diagnose a problem with his own breathing.

"It's using artificial intelligence," the doctor patiently explained about the spirometer, which measures airflow.

"Oh, I see," said Feigenbaum.[1]

Bed immediately after dinner was the rule for our patients. But not that evening. My office opened on the big center hallways. I could see them drifting in, silent as the bloated ghosts they looked like. Even to look at one another would have painfully betrayed some of the intolerable hope that had brought them. So they just sat and waited, eyes on the ground.

It was growing dark outside. Nobody had yet seen Doctor Allen. His first appearance would be at his dinner, which followed the patients' dinner hour. We all heard his step coming along the covered walk, past the entrance to the main hallways. His wife was with him, her quick tapping pace making a queer rhythm with his. The patients' silence concentrated on that sound. When he appeared through the open doorway, he caught the full beseeching of a hundred pairs of eyes. It stopped him dead. Even now I am sure it was minutes before he spoke to them, his voice curiously mingling concern for his patients with an excitement that he tried his best not to betray. "I think," he said, "I think we have something for you."[2]

From the time diabetes was first described by Arataeus of Cappadocia, it took nearly 2,000 years to the night in 1921 when Dr. Frederick Allen returned to the diabetic patients in his New York hospital from a visit to Toronto, where he had gone to investigate Dr. Frederick Banting's new drug, insulin.[3] How easily we forget what a dread disease diabetes was; but one day, we may look back in horror at video footage of people coughing and sneezing from the common cold.

MEDICAL BREAKTHROUGHS THROUGH RESEARCH

It took Banting and his colleagues years of testing on animals to isolate a single compound, insulin. In 1999, combinatorial chemistry techniques can scan for hundreds of thousands of substances at a time.

Is it any surprise, then, that in November 1998, a credible and respected American public television news program would report "dozens" of recent "breakthroughs" in cardiovascular disease research? Genetic therapies—which promise to go beyond insulin and provide a total cure for diabetes—took center stage. An example given was the bio-bypass, a genetically induced, protein-based method of encouraging the body to develop new blood vessels in the heart, thus enabling patients to grow their own bypass.[4]

The editors of *Science* magazine evidently would not have been surprised by the news broadcast. No fewer than six of what they judged to be among the ten most significant scientific advances in *all* of science for 1998 were advances in health care research, and a seventh was closely related. Following are the seven advances as described in an American Association for the Advancement of Science press release:[5]

1. *Circadian rhythms:* . . . a quick succession of discoveries shed light on how the molecular "gears" driving the circadian clock respond to light and temperature cues and how they work together in different organisms. The results showed a surprising commonality between clock workings in organisms from bacteria to humans. . . . These developments may ultimately provide insight into overcoming jet lag and winter depression.
2. *Potassium channel structure:* . . . researchers were finally able to answer an essential question about how cell membranes manage to allow in or out certain ions that are essential for sending

messages along nerves—the basic connection that allows people to see, think, taste, and touch. By identifying the structure of the channel down to the last atom, researchers opened new territory for understanding the roots of the nervous system.

3. *Cancer treatment and prevention:* Scientists added a number of drugs, including Heceptin, Tamoxifen, and Raloxifene, to their arsenal of weapons against cancer, and began investigating other drugs in clinical trials. Although the therapies each have their own drawbacks, collectively they represent an outstanding year in the war on cancer. . . .

4. *Combinatorial chemistry:* In 1998 researchers continued to stretch the applications of combinatorial chemistry far beyond the traditional realm of pharmacology. This technique, which allows researchers to make and test hundreds of thousands of new compounds at once, was not only used to produce new molecules for drug discovery, but also to develop fuel cell catalysts and other industrial compounds.

5. *Genomics:* The sequencing of several microbial genomes and the genome of *C. elegans* reached completion this year. . . . The genetic information will allow researchers to break new ground in understanding the evolutionary relationships among organisms and will provide a set of essential tools for future research that covers everything from how embryos develop to how to identify targets for therapeutic drugs. Researchers also completed sequencing the genomes of a number of harmful pathogens this year, such as syphilis, tuberculosis, and chlamydia.

6. *Biochips:* Researchers married biological research tools with microchip technology to create a flurry of novel micromachines this year. These tiny gadgets can do the work of many lab technicians at once, performing tasks including processing DNA, screening blood samples, scanning for disease genes, and surveying gene activity in cells. Major microelectronics firms have now entered the biochip business after taking notice of this technology's potential.

7. *Molecular mimicry:* . . . researchers provided the first evidence of a link between autoimmune disorders and infections such as Lyme disease or herpes simplex virus 1. . . . This development may lead to better understanding and treatment of a number of autoimmune disorders including diabetes and multiple sclerosis.

In this chapter, we will examine the source of these breakthroughs and consider examples of accelerated research; in particular, research based on computational models of biochemical processes. The computability of complex biological and chemical functions using the increasingly powerful machines we discussed in earlier chapters is starting to replace the messy, slow, expensive, and sometimes inhumane or dangerous experimental research processes and clinical trials of yesteryear.

By the year 2030, the accelerated research facilitated by powerful computers and related technologies will have brought us complete computerized models—down to the atoms making up the proteins making up the genes making up the genome—of entire organisms, including the human organism.

Gone will be the need for *in vivo* animal experiments that so many humans (not to mention animals) find distressing, and gone will be the need for clinical trials among humans themselves. In their place will be direct experimentation on computational models, holographically presented as solid, haptically manipulable replicas of individuals. The long-term effects of experiments and trials, which currently take years and decades to assess, will be simulated in seconds. And the researchers who devise and conduct health care research projects may be replaced by—patients themselves.

THE PROCESS OF RESEARCH

It may be useful to begin with a brief introduction to the process of research. This is partly for the benefit of readers not directly exposed to it, to help them understand this particular one of the forces powering the pace of change, and partly because of our basic premise that the accelerating trends described in chapter 2 accelerate the process—and therefore the products—of research. The products of research then feed back to accelerate the trends even further, and so the exponential spiral goes.

There is a third reason why all of us should become more familiar with the research process, and that is that we are increasingly becoming researchers, whether we know it or not, in the same way that we have become systems analysts: technology makes it easier and less expensive to seek, discover, and organize information and knowledge. For the moment, technology does not discriminate well between information that is valid and invalid, reliable and unreliable. Medical and health information in particular abounds on the Internet, and some of it is of dubious value.

An article in the *Journal of the American Medical Association* pointed to this deficiency:

> Judging whether . . . information is applicable and credible may present a greater challenge than just searching for information. To make this process more time efficient, Internet users may rely on a number of Internet resources that review and rate Web sites that provide health information. Theoretically, by relying on these ratings, users could more easily identify valuable information on the Internet. However, if the instruments used to produce the ratings are flawed (e.g., if they are produced to sell specific products or if they do not have any discriminative power), they may mislead or misinform health care providers or consumers.[6]

Several contributors to this book (for example, Brian Peters in chapter 10) discuss the rise of consumerism in health care—that is, the trend toward patient self-management, a trend empowered by the increasing availability of medical and health information on the Internet and the growing availability of home diagnostic devices and treatment kits, among other things. That trend will spur demand for, and therefore the development of, consumer-friendly discriminative research and analytical tools.

The process fundamental to both experimental and theoretical research in all spheres consists of the following four steps:

1. The collection of data
2. The collation and analysis of the collected data to produce new information
3. The interpretation of the new information in the context of pre-existing information to produce new knowledge and (when we are gifted or lucky) the production of wisdom in the form of a new or revised theory about how some aspect of the universe works
4. Disseminating the research and its results to those who are or might be interested

Thus, the process of:

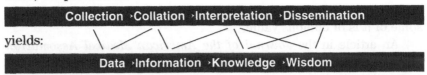

For the collection phase, we need to know what we want to know, what is already known about the issue, and where and how to find the raw data. For the collation phase, we need to turn the data into information, first by organizing the data into categories that can be inter-related in an analytic theoretical or experimental model, and then by applying statistical and/or experimental procedures to the model. For the interpretation phase, we need to correlate the new information with what was already known to produce new, revised, refuted, or confirmed knowledge. For the dissemination phase, we need to make anyone who might benefit from the new knowledge aware of its existence and give them the opportunity to access it, perhaps as input to their own theoretical research or for practical real-world application.

This process can also be expressed in terms familiar to the PhD researcher as the following six steps:

1. Establish a set of research goals, based on some perceived problem or gap in knowledge—the *research question*.
2. Conduct a *literature review* to find out what other researchers have discovered (and not discovered) about the issue at hand and how they went about it.
3. Decide on an *instrument* and a *methodology* for gathering and analyzing data.
4. Gather and analyze the data and produce raw information as *findings*.
5. Interpret the findings and draw *conclusions* about how they all relate back to the research question and add to our knowledge of the issue.
6. *Publish* a dissertation, journal article, or book.

If this sounds laborious and time-consuming, that's because it is. Or it has been up to now. But every step in the research process is now being accelerated through the application of new (and still accelerating) technologies.

Collection

The Internet, together with research-oriented intelligent agents, have accelerated the collection phase of research for both the relatively soft information that leads to the formulation of a research question and methodology as well as for the hard empirical data needed for analysis.

To keep abreast of developments and spot gaps in knowledge, researchers have traditionally relied on laborious, time-consuming, and expensive visits to conferences around the country or the globe and on the notoriously tardy process of research publication. Now, researchers increasingly rely on the daily delivery of e-mail telling of developments often a year or more away from publication by traditional means.

There are palpable dangers to the immediate gratification of consuming material so fresh from the oven it may not have finished cooking, of course; but to some extent the palpability mitigates the danger. Few people will venture close to the edge of a cliff, and researchers are generally unwilling to leap off one on the basis of non-peer-reviewed information. But they may be tempted closer to the edge.

The Internet is also increasingly used for gathering hard empirical data, which can be culled from public or private databases connected to the Net (which will soon enough include our healthcards) and/or can be gathered through written survey instruments posted on the Net (and, again soon, through verbal survey instruments built using automatic speech recognition software and natural language processing technologies). How soon is soon? Within five years.

Collation

Intelligent agents take care of much of the initial spadework of collation, too, by filtering out information not relevant or interesting to the researcher and categorizing results. This is particularly true of the breed of evolutionary bots that began to come into prominence in 1998, which learn an individual's information needs and interests over time.

Interpretation

The analysis phase is perhaps the most interesting in terms of the impact AI is already having and will continue to have on research. AI is fundamentally analytical in nature. Expert or rule-based systems bring the analytic experience and knowledge of experts to bear on a problem. Case-based reasoning (CBR) tools draw lessons from comparison with previous cases. And neural networks analyze patterns to aid in both classifying and predicting (drawing findings).

Dissemination

As the last phase in a four-stroke cycle, dissemination feeds back into the collection phase for new research efforts. And as in the collection phase, the Internet is becoming the paramount technology. It is cheaper and faster to disseminate information via the Internet than by way of conferences and printed publications, and the advances in machine translation discussed earlier are expanding the dissemination of research-based information to researchers from whom it was previously effectively withheld by the language barrier. The net effect (a serendipitous pun) is that more and more researchers have more and more access to more and more information in easier-to-use forms (such as ready-made data tables requiring no time-consuming and error-prone data (re)entry by the researcher).

The bottom line: More researchers produce more theoretical and applied research results more quickly, and that is why in the space of a single news broadcast we hear of dozens of recent breakthroughs.

Any and all of the technologies mentioned so far in this book can and do play a part in modern health care and related research. Virtual reality models and environments, particularly those with haptic interfaces, help researchers physically manipulate virtual objects from human bodies to molecules. The massive amounts of health data stored on millions (soon to be billions) of smart cards enable epidemiologists to assess and predict the progress of health issues across populations at any scale, with greater specificity, reliability, and validity than current probability-based methods can provide.

Extraordinary as such advances are, they are nevertheless essentially extensions of existing research capabilities. But there is one technology that represents more than an extension. It represents a paradigm shift; away from human-directed and toward machine-directed research. It is artificial intelligence.

ARTIFICIAL INTELLIGENCE

Artificial intelligence can be categorized into three branches or techniques: *symbolic* systems (better known as expert systems), *connectionist* systems (popularly known as neural networks), and *evolutionary* systems (with a variety of subtypes such as genetic algorithms).

Symbolic (Expert or Rule-Based) Systems

Symbolic systems rely on the fact that some manipulation of information can be achieved by manipulating symbols according to a set of rules—in other words, an algorithm. Few people any longer believe that intelligence can be fully expressed in this way; but for relatively simple, narrowly defined subsets of intelligence, then rule-based systems can do the job. They *are* doing the job with varying degrees of competence and success in helping diagnose illnesses and prescribe treatments, finding subterranean mineral deposits, and other tasks. And to the best of my knowledge, no intelligent machine has been sued for malpractice—yet.

The health care field was among the first to try to apply expert systems, perhaps because, in the first place, even physicians are prone to make mistakes and increasingly fall behind in keeping up with the flood of new research-based knowledge pouring into their profession. The vice president of drug discovery at Bristol-Myers Squibb was quoted in November 1998 as saying: "We can no longer rely on a person's individual storehouse of knowledge and experience."[7]

In the second place, professional expertise is (or was) hard to come by and expensive. If the expertise of a $200,000+ per year (and rising) physician or biochemist can be captured in a $10,000 (and falling) high-speed computer, and easily replicated to replace thousands of $200,000 per year physicians and biochemists, then it doesn't take a brain surgeon to figure out what happens next.

When symbolic programming—under development for only a decade or two—began to show real promise in the 1970s, what happened next was DENDRAL and MYCIN.

DENDRAL. DENDRAL took 10 years (1965 to 1975) to develop at Stanford University under a team headed by Edward Feigenbaum (considered the guru of expert systems, whom we met in the epigraph to this chapter) and Robert Lindsay. DENDRAL was designed to help chemists determine the structure of molecules, a problem previously approached through painstaking trial and error and relying on the expertise of the chemist. DENDRAL worked very well until the number of rules and logic grew beyond a certain point of complexity, when it became impossible to add new rules or make adjustments to existing ones without introducing instability. The system essentially became chaotic, with a small change in initial conditions having a large and unforeseen impact down the line.

Besides this limitation, DENDRAL was also an all-or-nothing system. It would only provide an answer when it was 100 percent certain of the correctness of its response. As we all know, in daily life few things are certain. This is undoubtedly true of health care; a profession that, for all its high-tech gadgetry and notwithstanding some diagnostic straitjacketing by payers, still relies heavily on physician intuition or heuristic decisions.

MYCIN. MYCIN, designed to diagnose infectious blood diseases, went a long way toward overcoming DENDRAL's shortcomings by separating the knowledge base from the rules governing when to apply the rules. Appropriately for a medical expert, MYCIN incorporated probability into its analyses. Its answers would not be straight "Yes" or "No," but "There's an N percent chance the patient has X infection."

The more fundamental advance represented by MYCIN over DENDRAL was the separation of the knowledge base from the control structure. All modern expert systems use this two-part structure, which facilitated the development of the expert-system shell—a control structure plus empty slots into which one could feed expert knowledge from any domain. The primary difference among the large number of modern expert systems is not *how they reason*—they all reason in pretty much the same way. The difference, rather, is in *what they know*. One expert system may know about infectious diseases, another about oil-bearing rock formations, and another about chemical separation through chromatography.

DENDRAL and MYCIN were important advances for AI scientifically, but they were not ready for prime time in the real world of chemists and doctors. They were neither big nor powerful enough, and the $200,000 professional could rest easy. For a while.

XCON. The program that counts as the first real-world, sustained application of expert-system technology was Digital Equipment Corporation's (DEC's) XCON—Expert Configurer. DEC sold minicomputer clusters that could be configured in hundreds of different ways. XCON helped DEC salespeople decide what configuration of hardware components was best for a given customer's needs. XCON then helped DEC production engineers put the components together in a cluster.

XCON helped make DEC profitable, for a while. But like DENDRAL and MYCIN before it, XCON too would eventually become bogged down as it grew in size and complexity. Nietzsche wrote: "The richest and most complex forms—for the expression 'higher type' means no more than this—perish more easily: only the lowest preserve an apparent indestructibility." DENDRAL, MYCIN, and XCON were "higher types" of expert systems, and they perished easily.

Other approaches were needed.

By the mid-1970s, other approaches did exist. By then, AI consisted of several subdisciplines: besides expert systems there were language analysis, knowledge engineering and representation, machine learning, computer vision, and logic. Language analysis was the forte of Roger Schank, who created a program that focused on the meaning in sentences rather than on their grammar or syntax. Grammar/syntax-based systems had already failed notably in the area of natural language processing.

The programs that Schank and his students and associates produced were able to infer meaning even where it was not explicit. One program, fed with news reports about the activities of U.S. diplomat Cyrus Vance, correctly "guessed" that Mrs. Vance had met the wife of Israeli Prime Minister Begin at a state banquet in Israel in January 1980, even though this fact was not explicitly stated anywhere in the news reports.

EURISKO. Making relatively simple deductions from a set of facts (creating information from data) was one thing; deducing whole new concepts from a set of facts—creating knowledge from information, something we humans are very good at—was something else altogether. But Ryszard Michalski and Douglas Lenat wrote a program that could do just that—learn, by example or induction, how to make new sense of things. Lenat's program was endowed with a simulated sense of curiosity—a drive to discover new things—and a simulated sense of satisfaction when its new discoveries turned out to be correct.

Lenat did all this in the narrow domain of mathematical number theory, but the key thing was the demonstration of the principle. After five years of dogged effort (supported, no doubt, by cybernetic reinforcement from Lenat's own curiosity and growing satisfaction), his EURISKO ("I discover") program was helping computer chip designers create 3-D circuits too complex for a human mind to grasp.

Predating the computer program Deep Blue's victory over World Chess Grandmaster Garry Kasparov by 16 years, in 1981 EURISKO beat not just one but a whole gaggle of geeks in an annual computer game tournament, in which human players control fleets of space battleships they have themselves designed in an attempt to annihilate each other's fleets. To prove that its success in 1981 was not just a fluke, EURISKO won the tournament again the following year, whereupon the tournament's chief geeks, deeply miffed, told it to go play somewhere else—it would not be welcomed back to the tournament again.

Significantly—and as Lenat has himself commented—EURISKO designed and tested its battle fleet in a manner reminiscent of the modern synthesis of evolution. That is, design and testing were accomplished through random mutations to the design, with a heuristic algorithm selecting or "preferring" only those mutations that conferred some benefit.

State of the Art in Symbolic Systems.   Previous chapters have included numerous examples of AI applications, including symbolic systems; therefore we will not belabor the examples. A single recent example will suffice.

Gensym's G2 Lab Expert is "an intelligent automated system for chromatography methods development and execution." By capturing the knowledge of senior scientists in an automated system, G2 Lab Expert allows process expertise to be shared across an enterprise. A novice chromatographer can use the system unaided, and since it will work tirelessly around the clock, the drug development cycle is shortened considerably.

It works by "emulating the actions and decisions of a separations scientist," says the company's marketing copy, and by "integrating liquid chromatography instruments, sample descriptors, experiment constraints, and method goals to develop robust separation methods and automate the time-consuming, repetitive task sequence of method planning, development, execution, and interpretation. Given initial run conditions and goals for the experiment, Lab Expert can reason about the results, determine the next logical step to drive the method to the desired slate of goals, and then execute the procedures."[8]

Lab Expert seems destined, if not designed, to replace the lab expert.

Connectionist Systems (Neural Networks)

In the late 1950s and early 1960s, while the superstars of artificial intelligence were pursuing mainstream symbolic AI in the form of the expert systems just described, Frank Rosenblatt of Cornell University was taking a different tack.

With a background in psychology, it was natural for Rosenblatt to approach AI as an exercise in modeling the human brain—which is, needless to say, a neural network. Before mathematicians McCulloch and Pitts made what AI philosopher Daniel Dennett has called their "modest proposals" concerning neural nets,[9] neurologists had been "desperately confused about how to think of the brain's activity. One has only to go back and read their brave flounderings in the more speculative books of the 1930s and 1940s to see what a tremendous lift neuroscience got from McCulloch and Pitts."[10]

Not only neuroscience, but AI also.

Rosenblatt's first effort, the Perceptron, garnered considerable press on the basis of its potential, if not of its science fictional name, but in reality it couldn't do much. The press of 1958 reported that the Perceptron could distinguish between a cat and a dog, but that was not true. It could do so in principle, but not—yet—in fact.

The Perceptron was essentially a blending of the concept of intelligent agents with the McCulloch-Pitts neural net computing function and the network learning function demonstrated in 1949 by Donald Hebb. The agents were photocells that informed the neurons how much light was being sensed. The neurons weighed the relative strengths of the light input reported by the agents. If a weight was higher than a threshold predetermined by the programmers, than a neuron would "fire." That is, it would tell the next level of neurons, which could light up pixels on a screen, about the light intensity. Eventually a pattern—such as a letter of the alphabet if words were the target object—would emerge on the screen.

Similar technology is now applied widely; in scanners, for example. AI, like the space program, does not have to succeed in the equivalent of landing a human on Mars for it to produce many valuable spin-offs.

Rosenblatt's principle, however—that neural nets could be trained to respond correctly to stimuli—was the foundation on which neural network technology was built, and many researchers took to it during the 1960s until MIT's Marvin Minsky and Seymour Papert (creator of LOGO, a famous program that let children concentrate on learning geometry through the antics of an on-screen turtle they could control with a mouse) published an influential book criticizing the Perceptron.

There followed a research vacuum in neural network development that lasted until the 1980s, and Minsky and Papert have been (unfairly) held responsible by the neural network community for the delay in progress of what was ultimately to turn out to be a fruitful approach for AI.

"Connectionists," wrote Heinz Pagels in *Dreams of Reason*, see "the essence of cognition as the response of a neural or electronic parallel network to input stimulation."[11] Indeed, the neural network approach to simulating intelligence has been dominant in AI since the 1980s. It draws its inspiration directly from the neural and parallel-distributed processing[12] architecture of the animal brain, and it is in the architecture itself that intelligence, knowledge, and memory reside—not in some external algorithm or on a disk or tape.

In 1974, Paul Werbos developed a neural network training procedure called *back-propagation* that not only overcame the Minsky-Papert objections but, it has recently been discovered, is a fundamental feature of biological neural nets. It is simply a form of iterative feedback—cybernetics—in which the results of the neural process are fed back to the network so it can learn what a "good" response to a given input is.

Back-propagation was independently rediscovered by David Rumelhart and David Parker in the early 1980s. By 1986, Rumelhart, James McClelland, Nobel laureate Francis Crick (codiscoverer of DNA), and others had developed this and other neural network ideas into a two-volume work long regarded as the bible of the connectionist school.

In the 1990s, connectionist technology grew rapidly and socked its symbolic sibling in the eye with notable successes in automatic speech recognition and autonomous land vehicle systems. But life is a compromise, and AI is part of life. The symbolic and connectionist approaches are now commonly used together. Each has strengths that make up for the other's weaknesses.

A major practical advantage of neural networks over expert systems is that they do not require much preparation.[13] An expert system requires that expertise first be captured from an expert and then represented symbolically in the computer—the difficult and expensive process of knowledge engineering. Neural networks, in contrast, engineer knowledge on the fly.

This means that it is much easier to apply an off-the-shelf neural network to a problem than it is to build and apply a (by definition) customized expert system. Several such engines are available, and the author has personally used an inexpensive ($395), easy-to-use, PC-based neural net engine with good results.[14]

Compared to analyzing data using standard statistical methods, a neural net is a breeze. Statistical programs are dauntingly difficult even to those who have had training in statistics—and in fact you really cannot use statistical analysis programs without first understanding statistics. Not so with neural nets. If you think you know what factors might help determine an outcome, just capture those factors in a spreadsheet along with some actual outcomes and let the network do the rest.

For example, you might want to classify people who have undergone screening for skin cancer into those who have benign and those who have malignant cancer. Trained on input variables (independent variables, in standard research methodology) such as skin type, results of blood test, and so on, a neural net can determine whether a given individual's skin cancer is likely to be benign or malignant.

Table 4-1 was obtained by running a neural net against a sample dataset of cases with cancer indicator data supplied with the program. As you can see, the neural net had a high rate of accuracy.

State of the Art in Connectionist Systems. Clinical trials of a neural network–based breast cancer detection system began in 1999. The program assists radiologists in interpreting mammograms and diagnosing

Table 4-1

NEURAL NET CLASSIFICATION OF SKIN CANCER SCREENINGS			
	Cases	Actual Benign	Actual Malignant
Classified benign	38	36	2
Classified malignant	12	0	12

breast cancer more quickly. Early-stage detection dramatically improves survival rates and cuts treatment costs.[15]

Hitherto, breast x-ray interpretation relied almost exclusively on the radiologist's visual interpretation. The neural net system can detect microcalcifications, atypical masses, and other early indicators of disease that might otherwise go undetected on visual inspection alone.

A different side of the health care industry is represented by a neural network trend analyzer that points pharmaceutical sales representatives toward "high-potential prescribers" and customizes the sales strategy for each targeted doctor. It provides "pre-filtered, pre-analyzed and projected prescriber reports to sales representatives in 20–27 days after the close of the calendar month," says its maker, claiming that a pharmaceutical client gained a two-point increase in market share for sales representatives using the program during what was only a pilot test.

Physicians may be interested in seeing how they are viewed, analyzed, and manipulated by artificially intelligent drug distributors; therefore, I quote directly from a company press release:

> [The program] enables a sales representative to focus on the top 20 high script writers for the last month. [The program] isolates only the high potential doctors in the order of importance, eliminating the time-consuming efforts of manually identifying who to target.
>
> [The program] lists physicians' script information by products and month. By looking at the trends of brands, a sales representative knows which brands are gaining or losing share. Armed with this intelligence, a custom sales strategy for each doctor is proactively designed, emphasizing the advantage of one product over a competitor product.
>
> By receiving [the program results] 20 to 27 days after the close of a calendar month compared to 50 to 70 days for other data sources, a sales representative can better track his/her sales effort. For example, if a sales call is made in the beginning of the three-month allergy season, and there is no feedback until 70 days after the visit, the season is over before there is an opportunity to change the doctor's prescription pattern. With [the program's] 20 to 27 day feedback, there are two to three chances to influence a doctor's prescription behavior during the season.

[The program] lets sales representatives take quick action to protect their brand against a competitive entry. It reveals which prescribers are defecting from their brand so they can develop aggressive strategies that reinforce loyalty.[16]

Finally, a health care–related example from the automobile industry: Ford Motor Company is applying a neural network developed at NASA's Jet Propulsion Laboratory to meet the stringent engine emissions standards of the next millennium. The network receives raw sensor data from a vehicle's engine and learns to detect and identify, in real time, malfunctioning components that contribute to pollution emissions.[17]

Evolutionary Systems

Evolutionary programming, the third of the three major branches of AI after rule-based expert systems and connectionist neural nets, was first developed by John Holland in the 1960s. It has itself evolved rapidly as a tool for modeling and researching optimization methods, automatic programming, machine learning, economics, operations research, ecology, population genetics, evolutionary biology, and entire social systems. Its techniques include genetic algorithms, cellular automata, and A-Life (artificial life).

An evolutionary program starts with the random generation of an initial population of individuals. Early evolutionary systems often depicted individual entities as clusters of squares, each cluster a random pattern on a computer screen. A simple algorithm (or heuristic) would cause the clusters to move around the screen and sometimes join or "mate." Each individual (cluster) in an evolved generation would then be evaluated for its probability of reproducing successful offspring for the next generation, and the patterns thus change, or evolve, over successive generations. Individuals with low evaluation scores would be less likely to reproduce, thereby discontinuing their lineage into the next generation.

An early and very simple example of evolutionary programming was supplied by Richard Dawkins. In the 1960s, he developed a program he actually called *Evolution* containing two subprograms, Reproduction and Development. Starting with some preprogrammed tree-like shapes on the screen, Reproduction would produce offspring from the parents, designed according to the offspring's own "genetic" makeup inherited from the parents.

The genetic makeup result was passed to Development, which determined the growth of the "trees"—their appearance on screen as they grew. Built-in random gene mutations ensured that, as in nature, the offspring would never look exactly like their parents.

The "environment" for (or "fitness" of) the trees was provided by Dawkins, selecting individuals for survival or elimination for no particular reason at first. This is a bit of a stretch from the not-totally-random natural selection that occurs in real evolution, but it supplies some of the randomness found in nature and now routinely programmed into cellular automata.

After developing the program and running it for the first time, "Nothing in my biologist's intuition," (wrote Dawkins in *The Blind Watchmaker*) "nothing in my 20 years' experience of programming computers, and nothing in my wildest dreams prepared me for what actually emerged on the screen. I can't remember exactly when in the sequence it first began to dawn on me that an evolved resemblance to something like an insect was possible. With a wild surmise, I began to breed, generation after generation, from whichever child looked most like an insect. My incredulity grew in parallel with the evolving resemblance."[18]

State of the Art in Evolutionary Systems.   Today, evolutionary systems are, if not everywhere, getting there. The following examples were contained in a comprehensive *U.S. News & World Report* article of July 1998.[19] It is a safe bet that a lot will have happened since then.

Evolutionary programming is being applied to solve complex engineering problems, find solutions to complex scheduling problems, and create complex new chemical and biochemical molecules. The word *complex* is associated with evolutionary programming with good reason: evolutionary programming provides a way to grow efficient structures too complex to be designed.

Complexity, though, can appear deceptively simple. Most of us have no difficulty accepting that a modern jet engine is a complex structure and would be hard pressed to sketch out an exploded diagram of one. Few Boeing 777 passengers, however, know that the General Electric engines that power their airplane were evolved inside a computer.

The aircraft's wing, on the other hand, looks pretty simple. Any of us is capable of scribbling out a wing design on the back of a napkin. Yet the fact that Boeing is experimenting with evolving wings for future airplanes should alert us to the fact that a wing is more complex than meets the eye. Stanford University is evolving a short-span, C-shaped wing that could support a bigger body and therefore more passengers—up to 600, or 44 percent more than a 747. The wing is so stable that the aircraft does not need a tailplane.[20]

The original human-engineered design for a prototype space-station girder assembled by American astronauts aboard the space shuttle in 1985 was "recast . . . as strings of numbers describing thickness, angle of attachment, and other aspects." A number represented a gene, and a string of numbers represented a chromosome. The complete "genome" was then replicated to produce a diverse founding population, and a genetic algorithm was run to evolve the population over succeeding generations. Finally, each generation was measured by the algorithm against a prespecified "fitness" definition. "Those that suppressed vibration best yet remained lightweight and strong were rewarded with greater fertility. Generation by generation, the fittest got fitter. The program threw occasional random mutations among the competing genomes to provide a little extra variety."[21]

After 15 generations and 4,500 different designs, a "lumpy, knob-ended truss" reminiscent of a leg bone emerged; a design no human engineer would have produced. Tests on models confirmed its superiority to human-designed trusses as a stable support. Satellite manufacturer Matra Marconi Space has contracted with the truss's developers to design an orbiting infrared telescope platform.

Employees at John Deere & Co., a U.S. manufacturer of farm and construction machinery and vehicles, enter orders for customized equipment into a PC. A genetic algorithm then runs through several generations of schedules and quickly evolves a final production schedule more efficient than any human—even one armed with spreadsheets, Gantt charts, and other sophisticated scheduling tools—could produce.

As if that were not enough, John Koza, a Stanford computer scientist who helped invent the scratch-off lottery ticket, is building a 1,000-processor supercomputer to evolve intelligent agents that themselves crossbreed and evolve. The implications of having such programs loose on the Internet are extremely serious. Short of a collision with a giant asteroid, there is probably no greater threat to the growing technological edifice upon which civilization increasingly depends than this.

Evolutionary programming is being applied in health care, too—in standard genetics among other fields. Maxygen Inc. used it to evolve a protein for antibiotic resistance in bacteria, producing a protein 32,000 times more potent than nature's own. Eli Lilly and other pharmaceutical companies use evolutionary programming to find new protein catalysts to help produce drugs faster. And Natural Selection Inc. is developing evolutionary programs that will read mammograms more quickly and inexpensively than a radiologist (and that will compete with neural networks that can also read mammograms).

OTHER TECHNOLOGIES

We mentioned earlier that any and all of the technologies and trends discussed in the opening chapters may impact research. Virtual reality (VR) is one of them. Like the AI tools just discussed, VR tools are becoming accessible to the layperson.

For example, one tool lets nonprogrammers create 3-D applications on PCs through "drastically reduced" development project complexity, in its maker's words. Users can create applications with detailed 3-D databases populated by entities exhibiting rich dynamics, behavior, and artificial intelligence. Giving ordinary users this capability saves development capital and frees programmers "for more involved tasks."[22]

At what point will such tools evolve to the point where programmers can be eliminated? Given the accelerating growth in computer power and in the evolution of AI techniques (including the evolution of evolutionary AI techniques!), plus the complexity barrier that leaves 3-D applications programmers facing a substantial knowledge, skills, and tools gap, that point is likely to occur sooner rather than later.

Virtual Autopsy over the Internet

An autopsy is a form of research. Medical students can today perform a virtual postmortem over the Internet on a Web site at England's Leicester University. As of late 1998, the Web site featured seven cases with information (such as patient history) that would usually be available to a pathologist carrying out a real examination to establish the cause of death.

By clicking on a specific body part—lung, body, heart, head—from the image of a body, the student can examine tissue from that area and then peruse and select from a list of possible causes of death. The list includes not only the right answer together with other plausible causes, but also some implausible causes. A right answer elicits praise; a wrong one, a rebuke.[23]

Three-Dimensional Scanners

Scanners are also turning into VR devices, with the development of 3-D output capabilities. In 1998, Japanese researchers developed a technique for quickly (in a matter of minutes) creating three-dimensional pictures from MRI images. CT and MRI scans produce only two-dimensional images, making it more difficult to see the extent of damage to the brain and the location of shrinkage. The technique was tested, with encouraging results, on Alzheimer's and FTD patients and is expected to facilitate faster and more accurate diagnoses.[24]

Haptics

Carnegie Mellon University researchers have developed a haptic device that uses magnetic levitation to enable users to physically manipulate simulated objects and environments in three dimensions on their two-dimensional computer screens.

Holding a joystick-like handle protruding from a bowl lined on the inside with six levitation coils surrounded by strong permanent magnets, the user can "reach into" a simulated environment on the computer screen and feel the force and torque of simulated objects. Its developers expect the technology to find applications in medical training, entertainment, flight simulation, and the interactive control of remote robots, among other things.[25]

The decade-old technique of "rational drug design," which used VR to design and build molecules to bind with proteins, failed to fulfill its early promise because computers were simply not powerful enough for sophisticated VR devices such as maglev haptics. A few drugs did result (notably the AIDS drug Viracept from Agouron Pharmaceuticals), but robotic techniques, which essentially merely automated and accelerated the traditional manual screening method, were to prove more cost-effective—in the short run. In the long run (that is, in a decade), however, increases in computing power and in the development of *in silico* research techniques have shown—as is the case with automatic speech recognition, machine translation, and other computer-based technologies that also suffered false starts—that rational drug design has survived premature birth and is maturing into a strong and healthy tool.

Database Technology

Computers are cataloging (collating) and analyzing (interpreting) the large amounts of data being discovered (collected) about human genes. In days, they can screen hundreds of thousands of compounds to identify potential new drugs. In contrast, traditional methods take on average 15 years and $500 million, according to the Pharmaceutical Research and Manufacturers of America.[26] (In that context, and even allowing for inflation, Dr. Banting beat the odds in coming up with insulin, but the point is still made.)

One company sells bioinformatics software for storing and analyzing the information contained in genes. A Japanese genome research organization offers free computer models of bacterial metabolism.[27] Such examples show that the move away from *in vivo* and *in vitro* experimentation and toward *in silico* experimentation is not just the stuff of the future but of today. What we can expect is accelerated change in the same direction.

"We're awash in data but we're starving for knowledge," said the vice president of drug discovery at Bristol-Myers Squibb, quoted earlier. Translated into the research process terms discussed at the beginning of this chapter, he is saying that data collection is no problem; collating and interpreting it is. Enter a company that claims to be able to screen 50 million compounds within a day. Only the best 200 or so compounds shown by the computer need then be physically tested.[28]

Despite the acceleration in the discovery of new drugs, it currently still takes years to test their safety and effectiveness *in vivo* in animals and people. That situation is primed for a major acceleration as increasingly powerful computers with increasingly inexpensive and easy-to-use software can simulate not just organs but entire organisms as well as the progress of any given disease.

In silico techniques have enabled the development of computer models of human and animal hearts, as well as the progression of such diseases as asthma and AIDS.[29] To quote medical science writer Andrew Pollack: "Using such models, scientists ask 'what if' questions, such as,

'If a drug were to block this protein, what would be the effect on the disease?' " Pollack points to the example of a heart model developed at the University of California. The model is used in the design of pacemakers, the interpretation of medical imaging data, and predicting "whether particular patients will benefit from a new type of heart surgery being done at the Cleveland Clinic."

Concern that *in silico* biology does not capture the full complexity of the body has prompted the Physiome Project, modeled after the Human Genome Project. Physiome plans to develop complete models of human physiology. Even if it can never totally replace clinical trials, it may nevertheless significantly reduce the number of clinical trials necessary and improve the effectiveness of those that are conducted.[30] It also marks a key step toward the development of the holographic, haptic, medical avatar DARPA expects to have ready in about 25 years.

Simulating a clinical trial requires the collection of data about drug absorption and retention rates, dispersal within the body, and effects at various doses. These data are usually collected from previous clinical trials and animal studies. An *in silico* model can be tested on virtual patients simulated to reflect the demographic, psychographic, and physiographic profiles of real patients. These include those who forget to take their medications. There are even techniques for simulating emotional states in virtual patients (and for reliably assessing the emotional state in real patients).

Glaxo has used simulations to determine what doses of a new diabetes drug to use in a clinical trial and also to satisfy the FDA about whether obese people and the elderly required special doses of Nimbex, a paralytic drug used for surgery, without having to mount expensive and time-consuming clinical trials of these groups.

In silico biology faces what some commentators think of as daunting obstacles. For example, they say, no computer is even close to being able to cope with the interactions among the 3 billion combinations in the human genome. Second, established pharmaceutical researchers may be prejudiced against the new methods. Third, not enough people are trained in both biology and computers.

2030 PREDICTIONS

In December 1998, researchers completed a nine-year effort to map the entire genome of the nematode worm *Caenorhabditis elegans*. This was a stunning technical achievement and a major advance for genetic research, earning a place in *Science* magazine's top 10 scientific advances of 1998. Many of the worm's genes (for example, the presenilin genes involved in Alzheimer's disease, genes involved in cancer and AIDS, and genes for making nerve and muscle cells) are also present in humans. The breakthrough was made possible only by the availability of computers to assist the researchers. The multimillion-dollar mainframe computers available to them at the beginning of the project were little more powerful than the $300 pocket computers available to them at its end. The human genome, with between an estimated 60,000 to 100,000 genes, is roughly three to five times larger than the nematode's, which has almost 20,000.

At about the same time the nematode research was reaching its nine-year climax, a U.S. congressional subcommittee was being asked to approve a proposed joint venture between Perkin-Elmer Applied Biosystems and the government-funded Institute for Genomic Research.[31] Perkin-Elmer planned to use a controversial new technology to sequence the remaining portion of the human genome, a technology able to load and prepare large numbers of samples of gene segments for sequencing around the clock automatically with minimal human intervention. It can take strands of DNA, cut them into segments small enough to read, sequence them, and then reassemble them into the original strand.

The project's backers estimate that "conventional" sequencing takes 8 hours of human labor for every 24-hour sequencing period, whereas the new technology needs only 15 minutes of human labor for each 24-hour period. They also claim that the remaining portion of the genome could be sequenced in only three years for between $200 million and $250 million. In other words, it took nine years and approximately $1.5 billion to sequence 20,000 genes,[32] and it is now estimated to take one-third as long to sequence five times as many genes for about one-tenth of the cost.

The Perkin-Elmer approach has been criticized for being less accurate than conventional sequencing, but that is not strongly relevant to the point I am making, which is that we see clearly in this example the acceleration in the pace of technology-based genetic research.

The spread of AI-driven research methodologies and tools, through the Internet and increasingly inexpensive computer-driven equipment, will extend to everyone on and off the planet by the year 2030. Any of us, with the aid of expert AI programs and haptic holograms of our own bodies, will be able to research what ails us—assuming there are any ailments left. In a new pioneering age, when more and more people will be living in colonies on the Moon and Mars or in space ships exploring the frontiers of space, there will still be the possibility of new and unknown ailments and injuries. Therefore, the ability to be not just one's own physician but also one's own medical researcher will be important.

As former U.S. Surgeon General C. Everett Koop and Intel chairman Andy Grove told a health care conference in November 1998, a power shift is taking place, with health care consumers getting ahead of professionals in embracing the Internet for finding and exchanging health care information.[33] Success in the health care professions and businesses will devolve to those who embrace the Internet along with other new technologies of research. Many of the companies mentioned in this chapter did not exist until recently. Although 30 years is not far away, neither is it overnight. Medical schools and research institutes have some little time to bring themselves up to date and give their students and researchers knowledge about, and access to, the latest tools and convey the need to plan on updating the tools at ever decreasing intervals.

It is amusing to see the doctors in the *Star Trek* television series wave a small device over a patient, which then diagnoses and heals the patient pretty much by itself. We will not, I think, pay someone $200,000 just to wave a $200 box around us.

References and Notes

1. Daniel Lyons, "Artificial Intelligence Gets Real," *Forbes* (November 30, 1998).

2. Quoted in M. Bliss, *The Discovery of Insulin* (Edinburgh, UK: Paul Harris Publishing, 1983).

3. See http://www.wiley.co.uk/diabetes/sample.html, which contains a sample chapter from a work on the history of diabetes by D. A. Pyke of the diabetic department, King's College Hospital, London.

4. *The NewsHour with Jim Lehrer* (November 11, 1998). Susan Dentzer's report said that "at this week's annual convention of the American Heart Association in Dallas, researchers unveiled dozens of breakthroughs that could make deaths from heart disease a

rarity again in the 21st century." A transcript of the segment is at http://www.pbs.org/newshour/bb/health/july-dec98/heart_11-11.tml.

5. American Association for the Advancement of Science (AAAS) press release at http://www.eurekalert.org/releases/aaas-sattra98. html.

6. Alejandro R. Jadad and Anna Gagliardi, "Rating Health Information on the Internet: Navigating to Knowledge or to Babel?" *Journal of the American Medical Association* (February 25, 1998). Article available online at http://www.ama-assn.org/sci-pubs/journals/archive/jama/vol_279/no_8/jrv71042.htm.

7. Andrew Pollack, "Drug Testers Turn to 'Virtual Patients' As Guinea Pigs" (1998), published at http://www.star-telegram.com:80/news/doc/1047/1:COMP34/1:COMP34111098.html.

8. Gensym's Web site is at http://www.gensym.com.

9. In 1943, mathematicians Warren McCulloch and Walter Pitts showed how it was possible for a neural network to compute. Six years later, Donald Hebb showed how a neural net could learn.

10. Daniel C. Dennett, *Darwin's Dangerous Idea: Evolution and the Meanings of Life* (New York: Simon & Schuster, 1995).

11. Heinz R. Pagels, *The Dreams of Reason: The Computer and the Rise of the Sciences of Complexity* (New York: Bantam, 1988).

12. Neural networks are also known as PDP, or parallel-distributed processing networks.

13. That is not to say they need no preparation. For an excellent and concise "how to" book about appropriate applications of neural nets, see Lionel Tarassenko, *A Guide to Neural Computing Applications* (London: Arnold; and New York: Wiley, 1998).

14. The software was NeuroShell: see http://www.wardsystems.com/.

15. The system, Second Look, was developed by Qualia Computing, Inc., and Briana Bio-Tech, and is being commercialized by BioChem ImmunoSystems, a subsidiary of BioChem Pharma Inc. BioChem Pharma news releases and other company information can be found at http://www.biochempharma.com.

16. The system is EarlyView, from IMS Health (http://www.imshealth. com).

17. Colin R. Johnson, "Ford Enlists Neural Net to Mind Auto Emissions," *EE Times* (November 17, 1998).

18. Richard Dawkins, *The Blind Watchmaker: Why the Evidence of Evolution Reveals a Universe without Design* (New York: W. W. Norton, 1987), p. 59.

19. Charles W. Petit, "Touched by Nature: Putting Evolution to Work on the Assembly Line," *U.S. News & World Report* (July 27, 1998), online at http://www.usnews.com/usnews/issue/980727/27evol.htm.

20. See the Stanford University Web site at http://aero.stanford.edu/.

21. Petit, "Touched by Nature."

22. NDimension Simulations' *SimStudio* (http://www.ndimension. com/).

23. Anyone can try his or her hand at an autopsy by visiting http:// www.le.ac.uk/pathology/teach/VA.

24. Reuters (July 14, 1998).

25. For more information on Carnegie Mellon's haptic maglev device, visit http://www.cs.cmu.edu/afs/cs/project/msl/www/haptic/haptic_desc.html.

26. Pollack, "Drug Testers."

27. Pangea Systems (http://www.pangeasystems.com/index.html) and Genomatica (http://www.hgc.ims.u-tokyo.ac.jp/service/tooldoc/ genomatica/intro.html), respectively. Genomatica is an integrated data management and analysis tool for genome sequencing projects supported by the Human Genome Center in Tokyo.

28. The company is Structural Bioinformatics (http://www.strubix. com/sbi.html). See Pollack, "Drug Testers."

29. Physiome Sciences has developed computer models of the heart, and Entelos Inc. has computer models of asthma, AIDS, and other diseases. See Pollack, "Drug Testers."

30. "Drugs brought before the [U.S. Food and Drug] agency in 1994 and 1995 required an average of 68 clinical trials on 4,237 patients, according to the pharmaceutical trade association, two to three times the number of trials and patients required in the early 1980s." Pollack, "Drug Testers."

31. Kristi Coale, "The Future of Gene Sequencing," *Wired* (June 18, 1998) and available at http://www.wired.com/news/news/politics/story/13079.html.

32. Coale notes that the current level of funding is $200 million annually.

33. Koop made his remarks at Intel Corporation's Internet Health Day in San Francisco on October 27, 1998. Reported at http://www.zdnet.com/zdnn/stories/news/0,4586,2156064,00.html.

CHAPTER 5

EMERGING PRODUCTS AND SERVICES

Cancer treatment and prevention: Scientists added a number of drugs, including Heceptin, Tamoxifen, and Raloxifene, to their arsenal of weapons against cancer, and began investigating other drugs in clinical trials. Although the therapies each have their own drawbacks, collectively they represent an outstanding year in the war on cancer. 1998 also saw an increase in public awareness of cancer, evidenced by a trend towards healthier lifestyles and keen media attention paid to some of the year's research advances.

Biochips: Researchers married biological research tools with microchip technology to create a flurry of novel micromachines this year. These tiny gadgets can do the work of many lab technicians at once, performing tasks including processing DNA, screening blood samples, scanning for disease genes, and surveying gene activity in cells. Major microelectronics firms have now entered the biochip business after taking notice of this technology's potential.[1]

C ancer treatment/prevention and biochips were two of the ten most important advances in science research in 1998. We met these and five other health care–related "top 10" scientific advances in the previous chapter on health care research, and I repeat these two because they are applicable to health care delivery also.

With more and more researchers producing more and more theoretical and applied research results more and more quickly, where does that leave the health care provider? How is the provider going to keep abreast of knowledge of the new methods and technologies, training in their use, and budgeting for their acquisition—and for their early retirement and rapid depreciation as more new and better technologies and methods emerge hard on their heels? Part of the answer will lie in the accelerating decline in the cost of increasingly powerful, complex (therefore, paradoxically, easier to use), and intelligent computer-based technologies. But this raises another important question: Who exactly will be the health care provider of the future?

Such questions will seem—I hope, by now—obvious. Yet unless one takes to heart the message of acceleration, one may miss the obvious. Consider this statement from the CEO of a company that makes ASR-based voice-control systems for operating rooms, speaking of one of his company's latest products: "The time to market has been remarkably short." What is remarkable is that anyone should find it remarkable.

We have talked about radical change affecting the health care professional at the giving end of research. We now turn mainly to those at its receiving end: companies that produce health care goods and services, surgeons, nurses, anesthetists, and other caregivers who use the end products of research to protect and enhance human lives, and consumers already beginning to use products directly on themselves that were once the exclusive preserve of the health care provider.

Which raises another question: How are governments, the health care professions, and consumer organizations going to keep up with regulating, testing, and approving the flood of innovations? The NBC-TV network's investigative news magazine *Dateline* revealed the practice among some eye surgeons of using laser surgery machines not approved by the Food and Drug Administration, with tragic results for some patients.[2]

To distinguish between givers and receivers of research results and health care products is somewhat misleading. I have previously argued that increasingly we all become systems analysts and researchers, and one of the arguments of this chapter is that we will increasingly become practitioners, applying the results of our own research and managing our own health care—with a little help from increasingly smart and powerful computers and computer-based technologies.

As with other chapters of this book, I present an exemplary rather than an exhaustive review of the state of the art. The following examples, taken together with others dotted throughout the book, continue to point to an overall trend toward total automation and designer health care based on the trends to smarter, smaller, more mobile and dexterous, more aware, more communicative, more interconnected, more autonomous, and more complex computers and related technologies applied to health care.

THE SMART ICU

In an intensive care setting, collecting and monitoring heart rate, blood pressure, blood flow, and other measurements for hemodynamic analysis is time-consuming and depends on the clinician's expertise to determine what, given a patient's particular circumstances, are acceptable vital signs and what are not. The vital signs of a patient in intensive care can fluctuate wildly, and it is critical for the nurse or physician to be alerted quickly to signs of deterioration.

The University of Pennsylvania Medical Center's smart ICU (intensive care unit) contains a neural network operating on fuzzy logic—a way of representing mathematically such vague and imprecise human measures as "almost," "very," and "quite far away." Fuzzy logic extends the machine's ability to reason heuristically, like a human. Instead of the plain heuristic "if approximately this, then probably that," fuzzy logic gives us "if almost this but not quite that, then maybe not very far from the other." Armed with this sophisticated method of reasoning, the neural net can rapidly and continually assess departures from a patient's ideal vital signs.

The smart ICU cannot—yet—get by without the clinician, however. In a 1998 study of 10 patients, the system merely monitored pulmonary artery occlusion pressure, heart rate, and cardiac output, and from this data produced 3-D graphs of hemodynamic status over time. One of the study's lead investigators was careful to note that the smart ICU was "designed to support clinicians, not replace them."[3]

THE SMART OR

Simply by issuing voice commands, which are then interpreted by an automatic speech recognition program, a surgeon can control an integrated network of smart operating room (OR) devices. A system introduced in 1998 consists of a set of interactive interfaces and a centralized control unit that creates a voice-controlled network of medical devices, including a surgical robot capable of positioning an endoscope in response to the surgeon's verbal commands. The surgeon can also command the endoscopic camera, endoscopic light source, insufflator, video printer, videocassette recorder, and arthroscopic shaver.

The system was designed as an open system so it can work with medical devices made by other companies. Its maker has reached agreement with a manufacturer of operating room lights, external view surgical cameras, and OR equipment-handling systems and is pursuing similar alliances with other device manufacturers in hopes of establishing an industry standard for OR control and avoiding the pitfalls of noninteroperability.[4]

NONINVASIVE SURGERY

In late 1998, German surgeons performed the first successful beating heart coronary artery bypass graft (CABG) procedure. The patient's blocked coronary artery was bypassed with another artery harvested from elsewhere within the patient's body and sutured to the blocked artery past the obstructed area. Since the heart continued to beat during surgery, supplying the body with oxygenated blood, cardiopulmonary bypass with a heart-lung machine was not necessary. Beating heart CABG eliminates the large traumatic incision and resultant risk of stroke and neurological complications, not to mention the long length of stay and recovery time associated with the traditional stopped-heart procedure.

The breakthrough technology in this case was a robotic surgical system consisting of three interactive robotic arms placed at the operating table, a computer controller, and an ergonomically enhanced surgeon console.[5] One robotic arm is used to position the endoscope while the other two robotic arms manipulate surgical instruments under the surgeon's direct control.

While seated at the console, the surgeon can view the operative site, in 3-D or 2-D, and control the movements of the endoscope with simple spoken commands. Movement of the surgical instruments is controlled via handles resembling conventional surgical instruments and is scaled and filtered to eliminate tremor. The surgeon can perform very precise, minimally invasive, fully endoscopic microsurgery with the robot arms.

The surgeon's arms and hands have been improved on with robotic arms, but the best arms in the world are useless if the mind controlling them cannot see very well. At the literally microscopic scales in which neurosurgeons in particular tend to operate, a tiny movement in the patient can throw off the surgeon's vision. Guy's Hospital in London has developed a technique, in working prototype and tested on seven patients in late 1998, that superimposes a scanned and well-defined image of (say) a brain tumor over the actual view a surgeon sees through the eyepieces of a binocular microscope. Image superimposition is nothing new; we see it all the time on TV.

What is different about Guy's MAGI (Microscope Assisted Guided Intervention) device is that the perspective of the scanned image is synchronized with the surgeon's visual perspective as the patient's head moves fractionally. In microscopic surgery, an overlooked speck of tumor tissue might make the difference between a successful and an unsuccessful operation. MAGI eliminates the need to clamp the patient's head rigidly, while ensuring that the surgeon does not (at least, not through technological failings) miss a speck.[6]

By reducing the rigor of surgery, MAGI will help make invasive procedures easier to undertake in environments less rigorous than the hospital operating theater. And so, too, will new anesthesia techniques: 15 percent of patients who received new, short-acting anesthetics while undergoing outpatient surgery as part of a University of Chicago study went home right after their operation, bypassing the recovery room altogether. "Already," according to a *CNN News* report, some 7 to 10 percent of operations are taking place in office settings, "and the trend is just beginning." CNN added: "It's too early to say where it will all end."[7] I disagree.

The Chicago study's Dr. Jeffery Apfelbaum asserted: "As with outpatient surgery, office-based surgery began with minor procedures, such as the removal of moles, but is quickly progressing to major procedures, including gall bladder removals, breast augmentation surgery, and pacemaker placements." Given this, and the estimate that today 70 percent of all procedures are performed on an outpatient basis, plus the trend to replacement of short-acting general anesthetics with even less traumatic local anesthetics,[8] then it seems clear enough where it all will end: in the patient's home, where it all began. The question is how long before the trend starts to impact the hospital and what to do about it.

The beginning of the end is clearly visible today in such new techniques as interactive MRI, which allows a surgeon to see inside the body, in real time, without opening it up. By threading an optical fiber through a needle inserted into a cancerous breast and having a clear MRI view of the tumors, a surgeon can direct a laser beam to heat and destroy them.[9]

In addition to the problem of keeping a patient still during microsurgery (a problem now potentially solved by MAGI), another practical problem in using MRI and CT real-time imagery for surgery is that the field of view is narrow—only a small part at the center of an image is in focus. Enter wide-angle virtual endoscopy with multiple-view rendering, which puts the surgeon inside a virtual cockpit with 180 degrees of sharp and constantly updated vision.[10]

It takes pretty heavy computer power to continually render a wide-area image in real time—the power of late-1998 high-end desktop PCs, to be more precise. It also takes sophisticated rendering software—the sort of sophistication now available for free in modern Web browsers: Virtual Reality Modeling Language (VRML). Here are the researchers' conclusions:

> We expanded on traditional virtual endoscopy by using multiple virtual cameras to create a virtual cockpit. The VC captures substantially more intraluminal area and displays it without the distortion that is inherent to many wide-angle lens systems. By yielding an undistorted 180° FOV [field of view], one can better visualize lesions that appear in the distance and examine them up close as they pass in view of the side camera. The VC technique affords views between the haustral folds of the large intestine and views of branching bronchi and blood vessels. Once created locally, the product may be viewed on a Web browser with VRML 2.0 capabilities.[11]

As of late 1998, the virtual cockpit was monoscopic, but making it stereoscopic is technically trivial. The main issue is the cost of providing the higher levels of processing power and bandwidth needed to produce two simultaneous offset views for stereoscopy, and it is beyond reasonable doubt that the necessary low-cost power and bandwidth will soon be available.

Even these breakthroughs could turn out to be short-lived as totally noninvasive techniques mature quickly. Consider the following three cancer therapies:

1. *Microwave therapy:* Celsion Corporation received Food and Drug Administration clearance for the use of its cancer-killing microwave therapy as an adjunct to standard radiation therapy for breast cancer in September 1997, though the system may not be readily available until the end of 1999.[12] In 1998, studies in the United States and England showed that used on its own, it takes just 10 minutes for the microwave technology to heat and kill an entire tumor and any nearby precancerous cells without damaging surrounding healthy tissue. Being noninvasive, the procedure eliminates the incidence of metastasization—the spread of cancer within the body—from the accidental dislodging of cancer cells by a scalpel or needle during invasive surgery.

2. *Proton beam therapy:* An existing alternative to microwave and standard high-energy x-ray therapies, proton beam therapy is already available at some 13 centers around the world. The technique employs subatomic particles—protons—to obliterate cancerous tissue. Massachusetts General Hospital's Northeast Proton Therapy Center, scheduled to open in 1999, will feature not just a more precise proton beam, but also a more precise way of positioning the patient for the procedure, using a new robotics control system that can manipulate a patient at the end of a 12-foot-long robot arm to within one-third of a millimeter of the desired position.[13]

3. *Multileaf collimator:* Yet another system has been developed to allow doctors to irradiate hard-to-reach tumors while sparing surrounding healthy tissue. Varian's latest multileaf collimator sculpts the radiation beam from a three-dimensional computer model into the exact shape and size of the target tumor, thus permitting stronger dosages (and therefore more effective treatment) while reducing or eliminating damage to surrounding healthy tissue.[14]

Medical science writer Kristen Philipkoski paraphrases a Varian executive: "Without a multi-leaf collimator, radiation oncologists must hand-pour lead blocks to shape the beam of radiation after measuring the tumor. . . . This technique gives extremely smooth edges to the perimeter of the radiation delivered, but is labor intensive. Plus, oncologists typically deliver the radiation from up to 12 different directions, and each change requires the technician to walk into the other room and reposition the block. With a collimator, the adjustments are made automatically using a computer."[15] One result, therefore, will ultimately be fewer oncologists and technicians.

Impressive though current techniques of minimally invasive to non-invasive microscopic surgery may be, the key point again is not the specific product but the trend. The techniques and products described could soon succumb to technological cancer and face extinction as even more impressive advances in health care delivery methods emerge. The trend to smallness lies behind two related advances that could totally change the way surgery is performed, eliminating endoscope, MAGI, microwave, and all: They are nanomachines and biomolecular/gene therapy.

SURGICAL NANOMACHINES

Huntington's disease, sickle cell anemia, schizophrenia, and deafness are among a growing number of diseases research is proving to be associated with the breakdown or absence of molecular machines in the body. Nanotechnology will result in machines small enough to be injected into the human blood stream to replace faulty or missing natural machines.[16]

In 1998, Princeton University researchers discovered that RNA polymerase, the enzyme machine that separates the twin strands of DNA during replication, exerts a force "equivalent to the weight of a red blood cell more than a thousand times its size."[17] The researchers are not sure how it works, but point to many other examples of nanoscale engines powering organisms at the molecular and cellular levels, such as the rotary engines that turn the bacterial tail like a screw for propulsion, drive the sperm cell toward the egg, transport chemicals during cell division, and reconfigure the shape of hairs in the ear for optimum audition.[18]

Another molecular motor, kinesin, avails itself of microtubules in cells to transport chemicals from one part of a cell to another. The Princeton researchers succeeded in making a kinesin motor molecule pull a micron-diameter plastic bead along microtubules attached to a microscope slide.[19]

Where nanotechnologists hope to build universal assemblers capable (among other things) of physically fabricating—from atoms—the chemical and genetic materials needed to repair or rebuild damaged tissue, biomolecular and genetic therapists might argue that this is overkill. Nature has already built the engines; we just need to learn how to use them, not how to build them. The first step in using them would therefore be to collect a storehouse of them.

It is possible to clone and store molecular engines. Researchers at New York's Albert Einstein College of Medicine have found in four genes the blueprint for the engine that drives the screw-like tail of *E. coli*. A clone of the tail contained the same protein structure as the original, which means it would function normally if attached to a bacterium body.[20]

BIOMOLECULAR/GENE THERAPIES

In September 1998, doctors at the University of Miami Diabetes Research Institute transplanted islets (insulin-producing cells) and specially enriched bone marrow cells from a deceased, unrelated donor into a 40-year-old female Type I diabetic patient. She was the first person to receive islets and bone marrow without receiving an organ transplant at the same time, thanks to a new drug called anti-IL-2 receptor antibody, which reduces the risk of rejection of the transplanted cells.

Diabetes is the fourth, sixth, or seventh leading cause of death in the United States (depending on whom and how carefully you read; the point is, it's high ranking),[21] with an annual cost estimated at $98 billion per year in the United States alone. How much is it worth spending, and how long will it take, to eliminate the disease and its high human and monetary costs entirely? And what then happens to all the researchers, clinicians, and physicians who make a living by studying, diagnosing, and treating it? The Miami operation will not of itself lead to the eradication of diabetes, but it takes a step in that direction and, considered in the context of the accelerated pace of new drug development, new diagnostics, and new treatment methods, diabetes' death knell has sounded.

We have already noted the breakthrough in CABG, and in chapter 4 we came across the biobypass, a genetically induced, protein-based method of encouraging the body to develop new blood vessels in the heart, thus enabling patients to grow their own bypass. But another method of fixing a broken organ is to replace it.

If the ethics can be worked out, cloning could be one way to provide everyone with an individualized organ repair kit containing inexhaustible supplies of rejectionless tissue—routinely collected and frozen at birth—for use in transplant surgery. Particularly valuable would be the individual's embryonic stem cells, which can develop into blood, bone, muscle, and even research cells.

The Roslin Institute, creator of Dolly the cloned sheep, was said in late 1998 to be in active negotiations with embyronic cell scientists, potentially including scientists from the University of Wisconsin, who announced in November that they had identified embryonic stem cells capable of developing into any one of the body's dozens of different tissues.[22] Apparently ahead of Roslin in negotiations is Geron Corporation, which announced in December 1998 that it would develop primate embryonic stem cells under license from the Wisconsin Alumni Research Foundation and Dr. James Thomson, who invented the methods.[23]

Among many other benefits, the technique will enable scientists to grow heart muscle for transplants, brain cells for treating Parkinson's disease, and spinal cord cells for injuries to the spine. How soon? There could be a cure for Parkinson's disease within a few years, the researchers anticipate. "The number of diseases that can be treated will increase exponentially [with federal funding]," Thomson told a Senate panel, from whom he was hoping to extract funding.[24] Given this development, the prospects of a long life for the anti-IL-2 receptor antibody drug look unpromising. Antirejection drugs would not be needed for rejection-free tissue. Indeed, the future of any one-size-fits-all drug, like IL-2, may now be questionable.

The customization of medicine to the individual goes beyond cloned tissue to the designer drugs promised by the AI-based pharmaceutical research discussed in chapter 4. Such drugs, based on a study of the individual's DNA, will save time and "bundles of money now wasted on ineffective treatments, as well as minimising debilitating side effects," said Karen Schmidt, writing in the *New Scientist*.[25] Schmidt quotes a geneticist as saying it will mean "a big improvement in the way patients get treated" and lower health care costs for society at large.

Pharmacogenomics and pharmacogenetics are the emerging sciences behind designer drugs and their future multibillion-dollar markets. The former "aims to describe at the genetic level precisely why some people respond well to certain drugs and others don't. Such information will be used to create diagnostic tests to help select the right drugs for each patient," wrote Schmidt. Given that "[a]dverse drug reactions caused more than 100,000 deaths in the United States in 1994, according to a recent article in *The Journal of the American Medical Association*,"[26] such tests would seem to be not too soon.

The expectation is that doctors will soon routinely test patients to ensure that the drugs they take really are the best for them. Biotech companies are already gearing up to sell genetic test kits to accompany the individualized organ repair kits mentioned above, and drug companies have already begun collecting DNA samples from people who take part in their clinical trials as a prelude to producing designer drugs, using another new technology: the SNP (single nucleotide polymorphism) chip, a microarray of common genetic variations in human chromosomes. Orchid BioComputer, Abbott Laboratories, Glaxo Wellcome, Genset, and Affymetrix are among companies already working with SNP chips[27]—an indicator that this technology, like many others discussed in this book, is more than mere hype.

Orchid's SNPstream microfluidic processor can screen 30,000 genotypes a day.[28] The chip is expected to help doctors identify patients' genetic variations to determine which drugs they will respond to and what diseases they are predisposed to. It will also restore life to drugs abandoned because of adverse interactions with other drugs or because a few patients proved genetically adverse to them—such as Seldane, which led to the deaths of six patients with a certain genetic mutation.

Adverse drug interaction is reported to be in the diabetes league as a leading cause of death in the United States, sending more than 100,000 people to the hospital every year. The SNP chip could thus result in a substantial reduction in hospital stays.

A counterargument to designer drugs is that drug companies may abandon the development of one-size-fits-all drugs, thus leaving unprotected those individuals who cannot afford designer drugs. But the promise of pharmacogenetics, given the acceleration in genome sequencing we discussed in chapter 4, together with the statistical comparison of data collected from large populations (aided by the smart card), is that any individual can be screened in the doctor's office "while u wait" and have a drug produced almost as quickly. Another concern is that this genetic level of information about the individual will lead to further discrimination in health insurance, with patients showing a genetic predisposition to serious disease facing refusal of coverage or higher premiums. Of course, as inexpensive cures and preventatives are developed, this issue will eventually go away in the absence of any other remedy.

Noninvasive to minimally invasive surgeries, nanomachines, and genetic engineering are concerned primarily (at the present time) with repairs to internal organs and tissues. Broken limbs have of necessity tended to be repaired or replaced with prosthetic devices. Recent breakthroughs in microsurgical techniques plus our increased understanding of, and ability to deal with, tissue rejection have recently opened up the possibility of replacing damaged or missing limbs with limbs transplanted from cadavers. Indeed, in late 1998 the first transplant of a forearm (with hand attached) was attempted in France.[29] The knowledge acquired through such techniques will be invaluable; however, evidence I shall present below and in the next chapter is that the trend toward organic transplants is at present being matched by equally startling advances in prosthetic implants, whether of limbs or internal organs.

NEUROSCIENCE

Increasing computer power through new architectures and better engines and interfaces has led to more powerful tools and metaphors for researchers and clinicians alike not only to understand and treat the brain but also to augment and improve it.

The U.S. Department of Defense is sponsoring research at Cornell and Johns Hopkins universities and at Science Applications International Corporation (SAIC) into hybrid information appliances, which the military hopes will lead to the manufacture of biocomputers and sensors to be grafted into soldiers' bodies and brains so they don't have to lug around bulky, energy-guzzling electronic devices. Rather than carrying 25 pounds of batteries, a soldier can feed his or her electronics on K-rations.

The technique involves building hybrid biological-electronic circuits using immature neurons that have not yet developed dendrites and axons, by placing the neuron on a silicon substrate and depositing micron-thin (1,000th of a millimeter) lines of certain proteins in a radial pattern outward from the cell like the spokes of a wheel. The neuron will start to grow dendrites (input wires) along the spokes. A dab of the protein laminin applied to one of the developing dendrites causes it to develop instead into an axon (output wire), and the entire neuron can then be activated by electrical impulses applied to the dendrites through the silicon substrate. The primary research goal is to help figure out just what neurons do and how they do it. Following that, the less militaristic researchers hope to see the technology developed into humane applications such as the regeneration of damaged nerves.[30]

Such research may be years away from success but not 30 years away; and even without going to these nanolengths, connecting nerves to electronic components at a coarse grain is producing results today. A 30-year-old government- and industry-backed project at the Huntington Medical Research Institutes in California aims to develop new treatments for neurological diseases and injuries. These efforts to date have led to approved treatments for epilepsy and Parkinson's Disease tremors and for restoring arm movement in some quadriplegics using electrical implants to stimulate nerves directly. Huntington is now working on implants to enable paraplegics to have sex and conceive children. Longer-term goals, through what is known as neural prosthesis technology, include restoring sight to the blind and enabling handicappers to control urination and artificial limbs with just their minds.[31]

As we shall see in chapter 6, mind control over objects is no longer the stuff of science fiction and magic trickery. Two patients—one with Altzheimer's and one with ALS—were able with the help of neural implants to control some functions of a PC by simply thinking about things they wanted the PC to do. The PC could as well be a robot, and the robot could as well be integrated into the patient.

Other approaches to building, repairing, and augmenting the human neural network are being undertaken by Professor Ted Berger and colleagues at the University of Southern California (USC) and Dr. Hugo de Garis at Japan's Advanced Telecommunications Research Institute. The 20-year USC project aims to restore functionality in brains damaged by stroke, head trauma, Alzheimer's, epilepsy, and other maladies by creating a parallel-processing network out of hybrid electronic/photonic chips that could function as a brain implant.[32]

Dr. de Garis is more ambitious. Using a chip called an FPGA (field-programmable gate array), he is seeking to construct an entire artificial brain with the equivalent of billions of neurons. The key advantage of FPGA chips is that their circuitry can be reconfigured dynamically. Using self-adjusting and self-learning neural network algorithms, de Garis's interlinked chips appear to function much like the neural network of the human brain.[33]

Much closer to practical medicine today are the brain scanning technologies of magnetoencephalography, 3-D electroencephalography, functional magnetic resonance imaging (fMRI), positron-emission tomography (PET), magnetic resonance spectroscopy (MRS), and the PET reporter gene/PET reporter probe. These machines do all manner of things, from mapping the blood flow and chemical changes in the brain to showing a video of specific genes in real time as they are expressed inside the brain.

Geoff Aguirre at the University of Pennsylvania has used fMRI on subjects immersed in a virtual reality world, enabling him to test a much greater range of thought-processing mind/brain activity than is otherwise possible for a patient pinned motionless inside an 11-ton magnet.[34]

Magnetoencephalography enabled neurobiologist Karl Friston to map a subject's brain activity as the subject decided to make small hand movements. The scan showed what areas of the brain were involved, and when, and (surprisingly) that it took the subject more than a 20th of a second between deciding to move his hand and actually moving it.[35]

DELIVERY AT A DISTANCE: TELEMEDICINE AND TELESURGERY

At the apex of the pyramid of technologies we drew in chapter 2—resting, drawing from, and dependent on all of the building blocks below it—sits telemedicine, which for convenience I will assume to include telesurgery. The federal government's Joint Working Group on Telemedicine has defined telemedicine as "the use of modern telecommunications and information technologies for the provision of clinical care to individuals at a distance and the transmission of information to provide that care."[36] It spans every echelon of health care, from first responder/emergency medical systems to tertiary medical specialty consultations and home care to the collection and analysis of epidemiological and environmental health data.

An example of telemedicine in large-scale operation was the U.S. military's Primetime III project in Bosnia. It provided 24-hour access to medical records, full-motion remote video consultation between theater medical units and tertiary care facilities, battlefront delivery of laboratory and radiological results and prescriptions, digital diagnostic devices such as ultrasound and filmless teleradiology, and medical command and control technologies.[37]

Telesurgery, a method by which surgeons will be able to operate on patients halfway around the world using datagloves, high-speed communication links, 3-D imaging, and cameras and robots at the patient's location, has advanced to the point where animals have been operated on from a distance of five kilometers and a human patient had a gall bladder removed by a surgeon from across the room. The main constraint on telesurgery is bandwidth—the speed of the communications link. The current maximum distance for a wireless link is 50 miles and 200 miles for a cable connection. Internet2 (which went online shortly before this manuscript was completed) is designed partly to find ways to increase the speed of the Internet so it could be used, among other things, for telemedical purposes.[38]

We noted earlier that DARPA is working on a five-dimensional total body scanner known as a "medical avatar." The scanner will produce enough data to enable a physician to examine a living, breathing, holographic VR replica of a remote patient, even reaching inside to feel the heart beating or feel a broken bone. It's about 25 years from production, DARPA estimates.[39]

Already, we have floating holograms of hearts you can feel beating in your datagloved hand, surgical glasses that superimpose digital images over real organs to give surgeons x-ray vision, and "robodocs" that assist in hip replacement surgery.

The message is that telemedicine is already here, albeit in limited form and limited distribution. Doctors use videoconferencing networks to view x-ray images or examine a skin lesion of a remote patient. VR already helps patients overcome claustrophobia, agoraphobia, fear of public speaking, fear of heights, impotence, premature ejaculation, and to control pain for burn patients and women in childbirth. Given the trends we have discussed in other sections, telemedicine is destined for spectacular achievements in coming decades, and the doctor's abandoned tradition of home visits will be resurrected in cyberspace.

All is not sweetness and light with telemedicine, however. There is policy to consider: policies ranging from "border disputes among professionals about licensure issues to concerns about the fiscal implications of more liberal insurance coverage policy."[40] There is, as Donald Moran also points out, "a healthy respect [among policymakers] for telemedicine's capacity to break the bank were it to diffuse widely under a regime of unmanaged fee-for-service financing." I'm not sure I agree. Telemedicine's wide diffusion would tend to be a result of its decreasing cost.

Telemedicine is also an indicator of the trend toward patients receiving treatment at home, as they did in the early days of medicine. Moran again: "In a world in which we can in seconds log onto a Web site in Tibet, is it rational to restrict the range of application of medical practice to the confines of narrow geographic areas?" I would add: Is it even possible to restrict it, given that the Internet knows no political or regulatory boundaries? If I hear of a Tibetan guru who (I am satisfied, after doing my own research) is a whiz at curing just the malady that ails me, via fiber-optic cable from his mountaintop, what's to stop me availing myself of his services? I would be upset if the government tried.

A further indicator of the trend to home-based health care related to telemedicine is the growing availability of home health aids such as the Lasette, a laser finger perforator that allows the drawing of blood in a nearly painless manner for glucose-testing purposes. The Lasette was approved by the Food and Drug Administration for home use, under prescription, in 1998.[41] In its own press release, the FDA noted that approval of the device could "improve the quality of life for many Americans who suffer from diabetes" and "[i]t highlights the many important ways that advanced technologies can contribute to our everyday health care needs."

HYPE ASIDE

The more I delve into such areas as health care delivery, in which I can scarce claim credentials (other than as an occasional consumer and a technology trendspotter), the greater my exposure to accusations of hype, ignorance, and inexperience. Readers with medical credentials are unquestionably likely to be more intimate with the specific health care delivery technologies I have discussed in this chapter than I am and may know them to be technologies that have not delivered on their promise.

Since I am about to embark, below and in the next chapter, on even more radical predictions for the year 2030 than any I have made so far, I must reiterate that the success or failure of any specific technological device is not the issue in this book. The issue is the trend or trends (to smallness, smartness, and so on) such devices represent and exemplify.

It does not matter, for example, that videoconferencing products "did not reduce physical referrals to a physician's office, but . . . required significantly more patient and nurse clinician time, compared with the controls which did not have remote consultation with a physician," according to a distinguished professor of medicine citing (in 1998) an apparently 20-year-old study of telemedicine systems.[42]

The professor acknowledged that "[t]he advantage could well tip to video links when video phones become ubiquitous. One could imagine many advantages to home care under that scenario." It is true that videoconferencing has not yet, even after 20 years of availability in various (and mainly proprietary) forms, become ubiquitous.

But the trend is unmistakably toward, rather than away from, video-conferencing. It has so far suffered primarily from a lack of bandwidth, but as the supply of bandwidth increases (and, as we saw in chapter 2, it does so exponentially), so too will the use of videoconferencing. Powerful image-processing desktop PCs are already here and growing more powerful through the operation of Moore's law. Enormous bandwidth is becoming available via cable TV channels and xDSL lines being deployed by the phone companies.

IXC Communications, for example, launched the Gemini 2000 service in late 1998. Gemini uses pure Internet protocols over OC 48 standard broadband fiber to carry high-end commercial and research-community traffic at a speed of up to 2.4G bps, 100 to 1,000 times faster than today's Internet. Full-motion high-resolution 3-D imaging—the kind of imaging that physicians really need and want—is possible at this speed. And this speed is already set to be supplanted by 10 Gbps OC 192 transmissions in the year 2000 and 40 Gbps OC 768 transmissions by the year 2005.[43]

The entire health care community should be actively anticipating the widespread adoption of high-resolution full-motion 3-D videoconferencing within, at most, the next 10 years, and possibly within the next 5.

And what about the next 30?

2030 PREDICTIONS

Computerized robotic surgical and OR control systems to enhance the surgeon's performance and centralize and simplify control of the operating room are available now. Enhanced visualization for minimally invasive techniques, improved dexterity for the surgeon, intelligent human-computer interfaces, and telesurgical capabilities are also not predictions for the year 2030. They too are now.

Realistically, these technologies will have shortcomings and may not live up to their promise in their present form, which will be seen as crude within 10 years. But there should be no doubt that the underlying computer technologies on which they depend will grow more powerful by orders of magnitude, and that this increase in power will transfer to these crude early technologies—which have themselves resulted from the exponential growth in computing power in recent decades. We can therefore look forward with confidence to more comprehensive and more effective minimally invasive surgery, improved patient outcomes, and a safer, more productive, and more cost-effective surgical environment, whether in the hospital, outpatient surgical center, doctor's office, or the patient's home.

Technologies will grow more complex, but the trend is fueled in large part and paradoxically by our need to make them easy to use—to simplify the end result. So, for example, complex supercomputers are popular among astrophysicists and meteorologists because they are powerful enough to translate astronomical amounts of chaotic data into simple and orderly visual images the human mind can quickly grasp. So, too, in medicine. "Before penicillin," notes Clement McDonald, "physicians had to know, and worry about, many different sero types of pneumococcal pneumonia and a score of treatment antisera. Afterward, they only had to know to 'blast it with penicillin.' "[44]

"One can imagine," he adds, "biotechnology bringing a simple cure or vaccine for diabetes that would eliminate the need to read whole textbooks about the management of diabetes." With the Miami method of transplanting islets into diabetic patients in 1998, we were beyond imagining almost as soon as the words were out of Dr. McDonald's processor.

Anesthesia will be so safe and simple it can be self-administered or administered by a robot in the patient's home. Hospital operating theatres will progressively succumb first to pressure from the doctor's office, which will become equipped with devices more powerful yet smaller, easier to operate, and cheaper than those that exist in today's hospitals, and then to patients' homes and roving robodocs.

The tissue repair kits and genetic test kits being readied today for use in physician practice will find their way into the patient's own hands by the year 2030, having become inexpensive and simple and safe to self-administer. Do-it-yourself (DIY) health care, heralded in the 1990s by the home pregnancy test and the Lasette, will have arrived.

Health care technology will go straight from producers to consumers, rather than "being filtered," as Donald Moran puts it, "through the academic medical setting." Societies increasingly driven by and beholden to free market mechanisms (which is to say, nearly all societies) may choose to allow the market to do the filtering, as is already the case for most other consumer goods and services.

In his review of health information policy, Moran also points to "natural limits on the ability of a stable or declining supply of physicians" to absorb the explosion of information on technological innovation, which in turn could "sharply exacerbate the degree of variation in practice patterns" already discernible among them.[45] Depending on one's point of view, this may seem less alarming as the number of DIY physicians increases. More physicians can absorb more information in toto, and patients' Internet-enhanced research abilities will enable them to fish for physicians with just the right mix of knowledge and experience for their own specific needs and self-diagnosis.

In the meantime, how are we to cope with the decreasing half-life of new health care technologies and techniques? As *Healthcare Forum Journal* regular contributor Stuart Davidson points out, the iron lung was the medical miracle of the 1950s and 1960s, before succumbing almost overnight to what he aptly calls "technological cancer"—the introduction of radical new technologies that devour and demolish the incumbent.[46] Part of the answer will probably involve a global used medical equipment market similar to the used car market, where wealthier owners (in this case, hospitals, clinics, and research institutions) will trade up to the latest technologies every two or three years, while their old equipment is sold to veterinarians and less wealthy third-world medical institutions. With much of the world's population still without access to basic x-rays, the market for used medical equipment is substantial.

Then there's ethics.

According to an article in *The Independent* describing developments in primate embryonic stem cell cloning, the researchers emphasized they had stopped short of creating a cloned embryo much beyond a week old, "thereby circumventing ethical concerns about the creation of a cloned adult."[47] This claim is hardly likely to halt the ethics debate in its tracks, but neither is ethics likely to halt cloning in its. Cloning, for purposes such as creating embryonic stem cell banks, is too valuable to human health care research and delivery, too tempting to greed, and too easy and inexpensive to stop. Thousands of small clinics around the world probably already have the resources to clone a human.

By 2030, all major diseases (certainly cancer, Parkinson's, and diabetes) will have a permanent cure. Remaining minor illnesses and small injuries will be self-treated by the patient. The role for those physicians still in the game will change to becoming bioengineers for those able to afford augmentations of various sorts—physical and mental—until either robots become smarter and more dexterous than any human physician (perhaps in human form, as androids) or the physician becomes sufficiently augmented him- or herself to stay ahead of the robots and androids.

The emergence of unforeseen new diseases and ailments, resulting from new genetic configurations and possibly from space travel, may still leave a role for the physician, whether human, android, or cyborg. Space medicine will be emerging as a major industry, fueled by a dramatic increase in space travel as technology enables ever cheaper space vehicles, colonization of the Moon and Mars, and the expansion and proliferation of space stations. The evidence for these developments can be found in NASA's plans for the next decade.

The hospital will become a high-tech body shop staffed largely by robots, taking care of repairs and augmentations which are possibly, in 2030, still too costly and/or difficult for the average do-it-yourselfer. Nurses and all other ancillary health workers will be replaced by robot/android assistants. Surgeons, too, may be replaced. Their arms already have been. All that's needed is to attach to the ultrasmart computer brain of 2030 the robot arms in use today for fully endoscopic, minimally invasive surgery, and who needs the human surgeon's eyes and brain?

"The patient!" you may trumpet. But the robot surgeon/nurse may well look, sound, and feel very much like a human; enough to satisfy the patient's need for a sense of the human touch. Those who will refuse to countenance such a possibility remind me of a scene from *Monty Python and the Holy Grail.*

A band of Knights of the Round Table, out questing for the Grail, are refused passage along the forest path by a cantankerous old man brandishing a broadsword. Casting gallantry to the winds, Sir Galahad slices off one of the old man's arms. But he remains defiant, so off comes the other arm, then a leg, then the other leg, and finally the torso; the old man defying the knights all the way down to his head, now rotating on its neck on the ground and shouting as they pass: "I'll get you when you come back!"

We have already cut off the surgeon's arms, legs, and torso. All that's left is the head, bravely but hopelessly denying defeat.

Or is it hopeless?

References and Notes

1. American Association for the Advancement of Science (AAAS) press release at http://www.eurekalert.org/releases/aaas-sattra98.html.

2. The *Dateline* program aired on NBC at 7 P.M. EST on December 13, 1998.

3. The remark was attributed to C. William Hanson III, MD, associate professor of anesthesia and section chief of anesthesia/critical care medicine at the University of Pennsylvania, in a press release available at http://www.sciencedaily.com:80/releases/1998/10/981019075219.htm.

4. The HERMES Control Center made by Computer Motion, Inc., http://www.computermotion.com/. The robot is known as Aesop.

5. Ibid.

6. Duncan Graham-Rowe, "Stereo Eye," *New Scientist* (November 14, 1998).

7. *CNN News*, 8:30 P.M. EST, October 18, 1998.

8. Ibid.

9. "Lasers May Remove Breast Cancers without Surgery," a Reuters report carried by *Excite News* (December 1, 1998).

10. For several relevant articles, visit the Radiological Society of North America (RSNA) Web site at http://www.rsna.org.

11. Ibid.

12. See http://www.celsion.com.

13. Massachusetts Institute of Technology press release dated February 11, 1999, available at http://www.eurekalert.org:80/releases/mit-sia 021199.html.

14. See http://www.varian.com/.

15. Kristen Philipkoski, "A New Weapon for Killing Tumors," *Wired News* (February 2, 1999), available at http://www.wired.com/news/ news/technology/story/17671.html.

16. Niall McKay, "A Baby Step for Nanotech," *Wired* (November 9, 1998), available at http://www.wired.com/news/news/technology/ story/16089.html

17. For more information, visit http://www.molbio.princeton.edu/ block/block.html.

18. Michael Brooks, "Nature's Motors," *The Guardian (Science Online)* (November 11, 1998), available at http://go2.guardian.co. uk:80/science/910790229-motors.html.

19. Ibid. Incidentally, physicist Sir Roger Penrose regards microtubules as a possible seat for consciousness.

20. Ibid.

21. Patricia Zengerle, in a November or December 1998 Reuters report entitled "Woman Is First to Try Possible Diabetes Cure," says diabetes is the fourth leading cause of death, citing the American Diabetes Association. Cell Robotics International, Inc., in a press release dated December 8, 1998, available at http://www.cellrobot ics.com/presrel.html#dec0898, says it is the sixth leading cause of death, citing the same source. The source (http://www.diabetes. org) says: "Diabetes is the seventh leading cause of death (sixth-leading cause of death by disease) in the United States."

22. Reuters story reporting an original article from the London newspaper *The Independent.* The Reuters report was carried on November 9, 1998, in *Wired.* See http://www.wired.com/news/ news/email/explode-infobeat/technology/story/16119.html.

23. U.S. patent number 5,843,780.

24. "Human Cell Growth Patented," a *Wired News* report dated December 9, 1998, available at http://www.wired.com/news/news/ email/explode-infobeat/technology/story/16730.html.

25. Karen Schmidt, "Just for You: One Person's Cure Can Be Somebody Else's Poison," *New Scientist* (November 14, 1998).

26. Ibid. Schmidt quoted from a *JAMA* article in volume 279, no. 15 (p. 1200).

27. Orchid BioComputer, Inc., gives a good summary account of SNP at http://www.orchidbio.com/mt_03.htm.

28. See http://www.orchidbio.com/.

29. The patient was 48-year-old Australian Clint Hallam, whose own arm had been amputated 14 years earlier. The 13.5-hour surgery was undertaken by an international surgical team led by Dr. Jean-Michel Dubernard at the Edouard Herriot Hospital in Lyon. The doctors followed the same procedures routinely used for reattaching a patient's own limb. The breakthrough in this case was the availability of new antirejection drugs, which lent the operation a 50 percent chance of success. A news report of the operation is at http://news.resoftlinks.com/980925/hand.shtml, and a *New Scientist* editorial is at http://www.newscientist.com/ns/981003/editorial.html.

30. Vincent Kiernan, "Researchers Pave the Way for Computers Built from Living Brain Cells," *The Chronicle of Higher Education* (January 9, 1998): A18–19.

31. Jonathan Weber, "Banner Year for Neural Technology," *Los Angeles Times* (September 22, 1997).

32. For information on the USC Human Brain Project, see http://www-hbp.usc.edu:8376/HBP/Home.html.

33. See http://www.hip.atr.co.jp/~degaris/.

34. Papers on this and related topics can be found at http://cortex.med.upenn.edu/papers_index.html.

35. John McCrone, "Wild Minds," *New Scientist* (December 13, 1997), available at http://www.newscientist.com/ns/971213/features.html.

36. The Joint Working Group on Telemedicine Web site at http://www.tmgateway.org/gateway/ offers a wealth of telemedicine information.

37. A June 1996 press briefing on Primetime is available at http://www.matmo.org/pages/bosnia/ph2press.html.

38. "Future Doc: One Day, Your Doctor May Treat You from the Other Side of the World—With a Little Help from Robots and Computers," *Fort Worth Star-Telegram* (January 4, 1998).

39. Ibid.

40. Donald W. Moran, "Health Information Policy: On Preparing for the Next War," *Health Affairs* (November/December 1998).

41. See http://www.cellrobotics.com/cell/presrel.html#dec0898.

42. Clement J. McDonald, "Need for Standards in Health Information," *Health Affairs* (November/December 1998). McDonald cites D.W. Conrath et al., "A Clinical Evaluation of Four Alternative Telemedicine Systems," *Behavior Science* (January 1977). The 1977 date seems too old to be true, and I suspect there may have been a typo in Dr. McDonald's paper—1997 would seem more appropriate.

43. These are just the base bandwidth figures for the OC standards. By applying modern multiplexing protocols, the baseband speed can be increased by orders of magnitude. Already, dense wave division multiplexing (DWDM) applied to OC 192 has produced speeds of 320 Gbps—32 times the baseband 10 Gbps of OC 192. Qwest Communications, a relatively new but major U.S. telecommunications company, had an OC 192 network in place and operating as of February 1999 (personal communication from a Qwest representative).

44. McDonald, "Need for Standards."

45. Moran, "Health Information Policy."

46. In an excellent series of articles on "Technology, Medicine & Health," published in *Healthcare Forum Journal* on various dates in 1995 and 1996. Most of the articles are available online at http://www.thfnet.org/thfj.htm.

47. See Reuters, note 22 above.

CHAPTER 6

ANDROIDS
AND CYBORGS

Cyborg [*cyb*ernetic + *org*anism]: a human being who is linked (as for adaptation to a hostile space environment) to one or more mechanical devices upon which some of his vital physiological functions depend.

Android [LGk *androeides* manlike, fr. Gk *andr* + *-oeides* -oid]: an automaton with a human form.

W e have reached a tricky point in an already difficult exposition; a point where we must countenance advances that are not only more futuristic than any considered so far, but that are so far from today's health care as to lack professional terminology. We must therefore resort to terminology from science fiction, which brings with it the risk of peremptory dismissal of the arguments presented in this chapter.

In hopes of preempting dismissal, I would remind the reader of the book's key theme: acceleration. The predictions made so far and those still to come rest on the thesis that Moore's and Metcalfe's laws drive eight technological trends that underpin, catalyze, and accelerate—exponentially—advances in health care administration, research, and delivery. The examples of today's leading-edge health care practices, given throughout this book, demonstrate that the thesis has been valid for the past 30 years and that it presently shows no sign of weakening. To the extent you agree with this—I think not unreasonable—contention, to that extent also will the predictions of this chapter be less of a stretch to your credulity.

In an age when low-cost home health repair kits and machines can detect, diagnose, and treat any common ailment, and when common ailments no longer include such difficult and protracted diseases as cancer, diabetes, and Parkinson's, then what will health care professionals have left to do? The answer is that they will make us better—but not in the way we traditionally mean. Health care professionals of the year 2030 will be occupied in taking us not from a state of poor health defined by the presence of abnormalities to a state of good health defined by their absence, as they have in the past. Rather, they will take us from a state of good health to a state of superhealth, defined by physical, sensory, and mental capacities not present in a person in a state of normal good health. The answer to those who would counter that we are unlikely (and foolish to attempt) to improve on 3 million years of human evolution is Viagra.[1]

The definitions at the head of this chapter come from my 1979 edition of *Webster's New Collegiate Dictionary*. Though dated, they are close enough to convey the meanings intended in this chapter. And by these definitions both cyborgs and androids exist today: people fitted with certain modern prosthetic devices are cyborgs, and the Honda robot is an android. In this chapter, we consider the sum total of developments in both human and robot engineering, beginning with humans.

CYBORGS

The same artificial intelligence–based technology trends that have led to surges in knowledge and treatment of the brain, which we covered in chapter 5, have also had an impact on knowledge and treatment of the body and our ability to replicate much of it. The development of a chemical- and bacteria-sniffing bionic nose was mentioned in chapter 2, and although it was not developed with prosthesis in mind, it could be. The same is true of an artificial tongue (see below). Other devices have been designed purposefully as prosthetics. Artificial hearts, lungs, and kidneys and prosthetic hands, arms, legs, and replacement hips have become almost commonplace in modern surgery. Factory-produced skin grown from the foreskin of healthy young circumcised males is being used for skin grafts, and artificial muscle is under development at MIT and other research centers.

So far such developments have been applied to the replacement of missing or defective body parts, but if they can be made to be superior to healthy body parts, is there any reason why they would not or should not be applied to the replacement of healthy body parts? And as we expand our exploration of space—a hostile environment for which the human body was surely not evolved—why would we not want to add new capabilities—never before seen in humans—and not merely strengthen existing ones?

I can't think of a single good reason why not. But once started down this path, where will we end up? The likelihood is that we ourselves will emerge as a new form of life. Our entire organic structure is set to meta-morphose, as a caterpillar pupating into a butterfly. Today we make arti-ficial human skin, bone, muscle, and blood, and we are set to be able to bioengineer whole internal organs from embryonic primate stem cells. We make artificial (and enhanced) sensory organs: nose, tongue, eyes, and ears. We make artificial limbs. And we are making artificial neural networks—brains. In short, we are already making artificial replace-ments for just about any body part you care to name, and we have the capability to make body parts not yet named. We may be close to resolv-ing the philosopher's question: What is it like to be a bat?[2]

Peg-legged Long John Silver might not qualify as a cyborg, but Campbell Aird, a Scotsman fitted with a robot arm and shoulder, and Clive Foster-Cooper, an Englishman fitted with bionic ears, would. These gentlemen may or may not like to be called cyborgs, but the term is technically accurate and is familiar to many people through science fiction books, movies, and television.

Many Americans, at least, are also familiar with a related term: the adjective *bionic*, from a 1970s TV series called *The Six Million Dollar Man*, which related the heroic adventures of a man rebuilt from electromechanical components after suffering a catastrophic accident. Strictly speaking (according to my *Webster's*), in its noun form *bionics* refers to the application of knowledge about biological systems to the solution of engineering problems, which is the reverse of what fiction-ally happened in the case of the Bionic Man, where knowledge of engi-neering systems was applied to the solution of biological problems. However, *bionic* was used in news headlines and reports about Messrs. Aird and Foster-Campbell and may come to be preferred over the term *cyborg*, which was not used.

Below are some examples of bionic developments.

Artificial Touch

An MIT graduate student was awarded the 1999 Lemelson-MIT prize and $30,000 for inventing an implant that endows the wearer of artificial limbs with a sense of touch in those limbs.[3]

Manufactured Skin

Apligraf is a bilayered (dermis and epidermis) skin "engineered" from the foreskin of disease-free, circumcised new-born infants and bovine collagen. Its use was approved in May 1998 by the Food and Drug Administration for the treatment of venous leg ulcers and eventually is also likely to be used to treat burns, diabetic foot ulcers, and sites where skin cancer, tattoos, and so on have been removed. Enough skin to cover six football fields can be grown from a single foreskin. The skin is effectively rejectionless—that is, a graft may induce, and eventually be replaced by, the patient's own skin growth.[4]

Artificial Bone

Biomedical engineers at Arizona State University's Center for Solid State Science are working on ion beam modification of hydroxy apatite, an artificial bone-like material, to make it adhere better to metal.[5] An immediate benefit will be to improve artificial joint surgery, such as hip and knee replacements, in which metal parts need to be attached to bone and inserted into joint sockets.[6] If it can be made to withstand greater stress than human bone, then it could enable a human also fitted with powerful artificial muscles to lift very heavy objects, leap great distances, and even—what the heck—flap artificial wings.

More down to earth, it would also circumvent the problem of bone loss that occurs in prolonged exposure to the zero gravity of space. A cyborg astronaut (with perhaps a pacemaker-assisted heart or a heart made from artificial or genetically engineered muscle stronger than original muscle) would have none of the musculoskeletal degeneration and weakness endemic to current astronauts upon returning from a prolonged space mission.

Bioengineers and associates of Rice University are also working on tissue-engineered bone, looking for methods to fabricate bone using a combination of biocompatible polymers, growth factors, and cell transplantation. They have demonstrated the fabrication of vascularized bone flaps for reconstructive surgery using formed plastic chambers packed with an osteoinductive scaffold and implanted adjacent to the rib periosteum in sheep.

Another method being pursued is to inject a degradable, polymeric composite biomaterial able to "guide" bone regeneration in people with skeletal defects. The biomaterial is moldable so it can fill irregularly shaped defects, hardens within 10 to 15 minutes, is as strong as the bone it replaces, degrades over time (thus avoiding problems encountered with nondegradable implants), can be replaced by new bone, and can maintain a specified minimum mechanical strength during the period of degradation and new bone growth.

Biodegradable polymers and bioactive scaffolds are also being investigated for treating nerve defects. Illnesses, injuries, and sometimes resulting medical or surgical treatment can often damage or destroy critical nerves. To restore neural functionality in a damaged area, surgeons may cut nerve or muscle from an uninjured location and attach it to the injured site.

Artificial Muscle

"The Artificial Muscle Project at the MIT Artificial Intelligence Laboratory is an effort to produce linear actuators based on polymer hydrogel. These actuators have characteristics similar to human muscle, in that they are linear compliant elements which undergo reversible length changes in response to chemical stimuli." So says the MIT project's Web site.[7] The University of New Mexico has gone even further than MIT, establishing not just a project but an entire research institute for the study and development of artificial muscle.[8]

Thus, artificial muscle can bend like a finger or lengthen and contract when stimulated by a simple electrical signal. NASA scientists are already thinking about creating hands made of such material for space robots, and it will be used to make "windshield wipers" for cameras aboard the Japanese Mu unmanned spacecraft scheduled for a 2002 mission to collect samples from an asteroid.[9]

Artificial Blood

As of 1996 at least six companies in the United States were testing partial blood substitutes in human surgeries. Not yet able to replicate the clotting and infection-fighting abilities of whole blood, the substitutes could carry oxygen from the lungs to the rest of the body and carry carbon dioxide back. Two of the products were to have entered final clinical trials last year.[10]

Artificial Eyes

A Generic Visual Perception Processor developed by the French Bureau Etudes Vision simulates and in some ways outperforms the eye. Input can come from video, infrared, or radar signals. Real-time outputs perceive, recognize, and analyze both static images and time-varying patterns for specific objects and their heading, speed, shading, and color differences.

The eye has parallel-processing circuitry around each pixel in its sensor array. Each pixel is analyzed by the vision chip with hardware that determines and scales luminescence, tracks color, remembers movement in the previous moment, remembers the direction of previous movement, and deduces the speed of the detected objects.

The $960 chip can be used for interpreting sign language, military target acquisition and fire control, and any other object- and pattern-recognition process.[11]

Artificial Tongue

University of Texas researchers have used MEMS technology (which we met in an earlier chapter) to create an artificial tongue able not only to distinguish between sweet, sour, salty, and bitter but also to identify the chemical constituents of the material being tasted. Artificial taste buds are made from the kind of MEMS technology used in the accelerometer of an airbag switch together with microfluidic technology—also the same technology used in the SNP biochips we met in the last chapter. The result is an array of what are essentially miniature test tubes, which are then mounted on a silicon chip.[12]

Bionic Limbs

Campbell Aird was fitted with a bionic arm developed by the prosthetics research and development team at Edinburgh's Princess Margaret Rose Orthopaedic Hospital.[13] The arm returned the use of his shoulder to Mr. Aird, whose real arm was amputated in 1982 to forestall the spread of a cancer.

The arm's complex of electronic motors, gearboxes, and pressure microswitches add up to a heavy mass, and it takes a lot of power to move such a mass at shoulder level. The development of advanced new motors in recent years has reduced the power requirement to feasible levels. The arm is covered with artificial skin: wrinkles, fingerprints, and all. Its builders estimated it would cost about $16,000 (1998) to build on a commercial scale for the limited market of people needing a whole-arm replacement.

But, it seems to me, the market potential for this arm, or others incorporating artificial muscle and bone, is enormous. It is not just a few thousand armless men and women, though it is to be hoped they will be the first beneficiaries of the technology. It is potentially billions of people who will want bionic arms for the extra strength and flexibility they bestow. The arm is also a major step toward a bionic leg, which billions of people will also want. Physically challenged folks do not like to be called "disabled," for the very good reason that they seldom are. In retaliation, some refer to the rest of us as TABs, for temporarily able-bodied. A bionic leg would literally put the boot on the other foot.

The most skeptical must at least concede that Campbell Aird's arm is a major achievement in robotics, and surely all can see the potential of robotics.

Bionic Ears

In September 1998, 50-year-old Clive Foster-Cooper was fitted with a pair of bionic ears, described by the BBC as "tadpole-like" and containing, of course, a microchip. Single implants, which restore up to 70 percent of hearing, have been available for over a decade, but this was the first time a double implant was given, the hope being to restore close to 100 percent of Mr. Foster-Cooper's hearing.[14]

Bionic Minds: Telepathy

Bionic brain implants allowing a computer to be operated by the power of thought have been developed at Emory University. A woman with Lou Gehrig's disease and a 57-year-old man almost totally paralyzed by a stroke were able to control the cursor on a computer screen and click buttons—just by *willing* it. The computer screen had icons indicating thirst, hunger, "Turn off the light," and so on. When the patient pointed the cursor at an icon, a synthetic speech program would voice the thought through the computer's sound system.

This seems to me to go far beyond leaping over tall buildings in a single bound; to be so mind-blowing, a detailed explanation is called for and is therefore provided in the box below.[15]

Bionic Faces

University of Louisville plastic surgeon John Barker has predicted that face transplants could be a reality by the year 2003. He notes that the knowledge gained from the hand transplant operation conducted in France (see chapter 5) could lead to transplants of the facial skin, muscles, nerves, and lips from dead donors. His remarks provoked an editorial shudder at the *New Scientist* at the prospect of a market among the aging rich for the faces of "The Young and the Lifeless." "Too awful to contemplate," said the editor.[16]

Perhaps so; but contemplate it we must, along with all the other possibilities suggested by these cyborgian technologies. The technical feasibility of restoring sight to the blind and locomotion to the paralyzed and augmenting human sensory perception to enable us to see with sonar like a bat has been demonstrated, not just postulated. There remains much to do before some of these technologies are in daily use, but the feasibility of all of them is beyond doubt, and so is the exponential acceleration in the R&D needed to turn the feasibility projects over to production.

Nevertheless, at least until we have developed the ability to give people a total body/brain makeover, we must continue to rely on external artifacts—machines—to perform tasks beyond the capabilities of our presently limited human frame and mind. The ultimate such machines are robots. Robots come in two forms: humanoid and nonhumanoid. We will examine developments first in the latter.

THE MENTAL MOUSE
Emory Health Sciences Press Release

Contacts: Sarah Goodwin
            Kathi Ovnic
            Holly Korschun

February 23, 1998 *[This is thought to be in error, and should read 1999— D.E.]*

Emory Neuroscientists Use Brain Implant to Help Paralyzed and Speech-Impaired Patients Communicate via Computer

Neuroscientists at Emory University School of Medicine who last year implanted a neurotrophic electrode into the brain of a paralyzed, speech-impaired patient, continue to help the patient learn to communicate by moving a cursor on a computer screen. Following the brain implant almost a year ago in March 1998, the patient first learned to express himself by indicating phrases on the computer screen such as "I am thirsty" and "It was nice talking to you." More recently he has learned to move the cursor to letters of the alphabet and spell his own name and the name of his doctors.

Roy A. E. Bakay, MD, a neurosurgeon at Emory University School of Medicine and neurologist Philip R. Kennedy, MD, developed the neurotrophic electrode, which they first implanted in 1997 in a woman who was "locked in" and unable to speak due to amyotrophic lateral sclerosis (ALS, or Lou Gehrig's disease). At the time of her death from ALS, the patient was learning to control the neural signals from her implant. Results from this research were published in the June 1998 issue of *NeuroReport*.

Last year the Emory physicians implanted an electrode into the brain of a patient who is paralyzed from the neck down and has been unable to speak since a brainstem stroke late in 1997. The patient is at the Emory-affiliated Atlanta Veterans Affairs Medical Center and has been learning to use a computer over the past few months to communicate with simple phrases and letters. Dr. Kennedy likens the technology to "a mental mouse" that allows the patient to move the cursor as if he held a computer mouse in his hand.

Drs. Kennedy and Bakay are hopeful that the new technology will eventually progress to the point where patients will be able to communicate smoothly and accomplish tasks such as turning on light switches and sending e-mail.

"A person can interact with the world if they can use a computer," Dr. Bakay said. "This development will open up a tremendous amount of opportunity for patients who have lost the ability to move and talk because of stroke, spinal cord injury or diseases like Lou Gehrig's disease."

(Continued on next page)

THE MENTAL MOUSE
Emory Health Sciences Press Release (Continued)

The neurotrophic electrode is implanted into the motor cortex of the brain using a tiny glass encasing. Neurotrophic growth factors are implanted into the glass, and the cortical cells grow into the electrode and form neural contacts. It takes several weeks for the cortical tissue to grow into the electrode.

The neurons in the brain transmit an electronic signal when they "fire." Recording wires placed inside the glass cone pick up the neural signals from the ingrown brain tissue and transmit then through the skin to a receiver and amplifier outside of the scalp. The system is powered by an induction coil placed over the scalp. There are no wires going through the skin. The recorded neural signals are connected to the computer and are used as a substitute for the mouse cursor. The patient is able to hear noises that indicate when his brain is thinking in a way that will allow him to focus on the cursor and move it.

"The trick is teaching the patient to control the strength and pattern of the electric impulses being produced in the brain," Dr. Bakay said. "After some training, the patient is able to 'will' a cursor to move and then stop on a specific point on the computer screen."

"This new technique has profound implications for paralyzed people everywhere, whether paralyzed by spinal cord or brainstem injury, or by such devastating diseases as ALS," Dr. Kennedy says. "For spinal cord injured patients who have uncontrolled muscles, these neural signals could provide some control of electrical stimulators that activate the paralyzed muscles, thus bypassing the area of spinal cord injury ("spinal bypass"). Right now we are concentrating our efforts on the relatively easier task of providing a communication link to a computer for locked-in patients."

NONHUMANOID ROBOTS

Autonomous robots are the ultimate in augmentative and labor-saving extensions to our limited human capabilities. We have already met the soft variety—bots and agents, which do their work in cyberspace. Now we are talking about their hardware cousins, which work in physical space. Robots of both varieties do the work they are designed to do without any instruction beyond their initial, built-in programs. One of the first things we want them to do is to stop pestering us for help, maintenance, and instructions. A robot that can do the work of 10 people at a tenth of the price of one is not such a big deal if it takes 20 people to control and maintain it.

To work autonomously does not necessarily mean that a robot must be detached from the rest of the world, but in many cases they are. Suppose you wanted (and Hugo de Garis, the researcher trying to build a kitten brain out of FPGA chips in Japan, is already working on it) a vacuum cleaner that would roam the house or the hospital on its own, cleaning as it goes, and whistling a happy tune. It could be connected to its energy source (the electrical supply) with a cord, as is usually the case today, but it would be more convenient if it were cordless. That means it must run on batteries, and that means the batteries will need charging—the robot will need to eat.

Scott Jantz and Keith L. Doty of the Machine Intelligence Laboratory at the University of Florida have taught robots to eat—to find a battery charger and plug in when their batteries run low. They endowed their robots with a learning algorithm that would let the robots figure out their own eating habits. The robots learned to stay in the most efficient region of the batteries' operation. In other words, they learned to eat wisely: not so little that they would run out of steam in the middle of a job, and not so gluttonously that they would waste energy.

The scientists also gave their progeny a realistic environment in the sense that their food resources (battery chargers) were not unlimited, and they had to compete for their dinners. Those that did not compete successfully ran out of juice and "died."

But the ultimate goal of the research was not a feeding robot. During the 1950s a vacuum-tube robot "turtle" built by W. Grey Walter could already recharge itself, and, besides, within the next decade we will see self-charging, self-contained power units eliminate today's inadequate, overpriced, and environmentally disreputable batteries. German researchers have already produced a hydrogen fuel cell small enough to fit in a laptop computer.[17]

Jantz and Doty's main goal, however, was much more important than extended battery life. Rather, it was "to develop a robust robotic platform capable of surviving for an indefinite period of time without human intervention. Learning algorithms are implemented in the agents to facilitate the longevity of the robots and to imbue the robots with a primitive instinct for survival."

In 1998, a German-made autonomous tour-guide/tutor robot helped visitors to the Deutsches Museum in Bonn and, later in the year at the Smithsonian in Washington, find their way to exhibits and (if desired) explain the exhibit. The robot could navigate at walking speed through dense crowds while reliably avoiding collisions with obstacles. Its developers argue that the "time is ripe for the development of AI-based commercial service robots that assist people in everyday life."[18]

If you find a little unsettling the notion of a powerful, smart, and untethered robot able to get along just fine without human help, thank you—then wait, there's more. Professor Doty and colleague Ronald E. Van Aken in 1993 created a software simulation (an Alife program) of a swarm of robots whose emergent behavior successfully performed the required activities without central planning. Swarm robots are "groups of autonomous mobile robots whose sensory-driven state behavior produces emergent group functionality not characteristic of the individual robots," they wrote, meaning that the robots have a natural tendency to gang up.[19]

The swarm robots had sensors to detect collisions with one another, walls, and other elements in the environment. "The sensors served as inputs to robot state machine controls and essentially allowed the robot to adapt and interact with its environment without learning." There was, however, a level of command and control, and we'll get to that in a moment. Meanwhile, the Johns Hopkins University (JHU) Robotics Lab has been busy building robot swarms—this time in hardware—that can join together in various configurations, rather like constructor toys that can change shape and function—with a little help from the kids.

They are called *metamorphic* robots. "A Metamorphic Robotic System," says JHU's Web site, "is a collection of independently controlled mechatronic modules, each of which has the ability to connect, disconnect and climb over adjacent modules. Each module allows power and information to flow through itself and to its neighbors. A change in manipulator morphology results from the locomotion of each module over its neighbors. Thus a metamorphic system has the ability to dynamically reconfigure."[20]

Putting it all together, what we have so far is a bunch of creepy but lovable little monsters able to do their own thing, feed themselves, gang up to fight for survival, and metamorphose if needed. Their "thing" is to some extent preprogrammed (into the individual robots), but at a higher level various behaviors just emerge when they get together. This is not so far removed, in principle, from a description of an ant colony. Some ant species are known to clump together and "metamorphose" into a bridge to enable their colleagues to cross an ant ravine. Thankfully, neither ants nor our metamorphic swarm robots are very big, power-ful, armed, or smart. Yet.

But as for smart, re-enter Professor Doty, this time with IBM researcher Akram Bou-Ghannam in tow. Together, they have worked on the control architecture for an intelligent, fully autonomous, mobile robot.

Noting that "[a]nimals live in a dynamic environment and tailor their actions based on their internal state and their perception of the external environment," and that "[a]nimal interaction with the environment becomes more complex as one ascends the hierarchy of organisms," they conclude that "[a]nimals lower in the hierarchy behave reactively to stimuli where those at the top end of the hierarchy employ learning and intelligence."[21]

This is much in line with the hypothesis that lower-order animals rely more on basic (instinctual, hard-wired, algorithmic, preprogrammed, mimoemorphic) decisions than on acquired decisions (basic decisions refined through heuristics in response to experience), and even less (if at all) on intellectual (strictly memetic, polimorphic) decisions.[22]

The question for Doty and Bou-Ghannam, then, was: Should robots be modeled on human behavior and intelligence that relies more on intellect, or on insect-like intelligence that relies on basic, instinctual behaviors? Their answer was to combine both, but since humans already combine intellect with basic, instinctual intelligence, then to my mind they really opted for the human model.

The three principal components of the Doty/Bou-Ghannam robot were: (1) A *behavior* component, essentially a set of preprogrammed algorithmic responses to stimuli—the hard-wiring; (2) a *perceptual* component, consisting of sensors and programs that perform initial heuristic processing of sensory input and pass it to the cognitive component for analysis, integration with previous knowledge, and, if necessary, instructions to the behavioral component that controls the robot's actions; and (3) a *cognitive* component, which manipulates perceptual knowledge representations and performs higher machine intelligence functions such as planning.

Through cybernetic feedback and feedforward loops similar to those in the human body, the three components are constantly letting one another know what is going on in their neck of the woods. A key aspect of the processing is that it occurs in parallel. Parallel processing, as we saw in chapter 2, is well known to the computing world as a means of gaining quantum jumps in processing speed over traditional serial processing, and it is the way the human body's neural network operates.

The Doty robots are not the most beautiful of creations, and they currently don't do much at all beyond mooch around a lab. They are a bunch of wires, motors, computer chips, and so forth sitting atop circular metal plates with wheels on the bottom. Philosophically, they may or may not turn out to be monsters when they grow up, but the chances are they won't look like monsters. Chances are they may look remarkably like you and me if they are designed as general purpose robots as opposed to special-function robots.

ANDROIDS

Also known as humanoid robots, androids as human-like in physical appearance as Commander Data in the *Star Trek: The Next Generation* TV series may be closer than you think. Skin made up of fabric with thousands of tiny touch-sensitive transducers woven into each square inch will cover their limbs. Such fabric is already used for data gloves and data suits in virtual reality environments requiring tactile sensations and haptic feedback. Later, it will probably be possible and could be less expensive to give them the real skin we discussed earlier.

The limbs of future humanoid robots may not be the clanking mess of solenoids, rods, motors, nuts, and bolts of today's robots (and Campbell Aird's arm) but be made of materials much like human tissues, such as the artificial muscle we also met earlier.

The Mark I of all true androids is the Honda robot. Previous versions have been toys, ornaments, or prototypes, but the Honda really works. It has some way to go in the finer details of its human form, but it satisfies *Webster's* and is more like a human than it is like anything else. Where Honda shines in the locomotive aspects of androidism, its American cousin Cog shines in the cognitive aspects.[23]

Recall from chapter 2 that Cog does not even have legs to walk on, yet. It has a head, with brain, eyes, and ears; and it has a torso with two arms and hands. Legs can always be retrofitted. Rodney Brooks would rather have his creation understand and be able to interact with the world before letting it make its own bipedal way therein. Which makes a lot of sense. It would not do to have newborn human infants running, walking, or even crawling around until they have assimilated some basic physical realities, such as the laws of gravity and thermodynamics at a rudimentary survival level.

Brooks is therefore focusing on teaching Cog to coordinate its eye, head, and hand movements. He is convinced that letting a machine discover the world on its own the way humans do rather than preprogramming its memory with facts is the most efficient and the fastest approach to true AI.

By the summer of 1996, Cog was reacting to its environment in a manner realistic enough to make people react to it as though it were human (shades of Eliza, the psychotherapy program that fools many people into thinking it is a real person). The intention was to add sensory capabilities, including touch and smell, bit by bit, and just two years since that summer an artificial nose and tongue have become available for it, if Brooks wishes.

2030 PREDICTIONS

Traditional health insurance may be meaningless in an age when normal good health is ensured (not just insured) cheaply for virtually everyone. Good health, as we know it today, will come cheap and will be perceived as a fundamental human right. Superhealth will not; at least, not initially. The initial recipients of total body makeovers will be specialist soldiers and police, astronauts, entertainers, the rich, and health care professionals themselves.

Health insurance might change to something more akin to auto or homeowners insurance with provisions for collision damage and disaster coverage, probably with deductibles and higher premiums for the accident-prone and high-risk takers such as early space travelers. Like a luxury car, the more augmented the individual—the more bells, whistles, and exotic materials—the higher the cost of insurance.

Cyborg technology will continue to accelerate, and people will want to upgrade themselves at regular intervals. Much of the work involved in reengineering people as cyborgs will be done by robots, by cyborg physicians, or (most likely) by both, acting as a team.

The Holy Grail of nanotechnology, the universal assembler, will play an increasing (and ultimately the solo) role in cyboengineering.

The human body may become a mix of hardware and biological "wetware." So too might some android bodies, to the extent that cyborgs and humans could become indistinguishable. Certain wetware functions may turn out to be optimal (as opposed to hardware alternatives), at least for life on Earth. For those who leave Earth forever to explore the universe, an all-hardware body may be more robust. Roboticist Hans Moravec has proposed the concept of downloading human minds into android bodies for long-range space travel.

Human sexual urges may well be satisfied to a large extent through machines, but nature will keep a watchful eye on our reproductive needs as a (new) species. Cloning of whole individuals will not be the answer because evolutionary progress demands diversity, not uniformity.

Don't forget that radio, TV, telephone, automobile, airplane, rocket ship, submarine, and the x-ray were all science fiction once.

References and Notes

1. There may be ethical and/or long-term scientific reasons for discounting Viagra's contribution to a state of superhealth, but for the here and now, and for better or worse, society—through the market—has spoken quite decisively.

2. Philosopher Thomas Nagel published a much-discussed essay, "What Is It Like to Be a Bat?" in *The Philosophical Review* (October 1974). It was reprinted in Douglas R. Hofstadter and D. C. Dennett, eds., *The Mind's I: Fantasies and Reflections on Self and Soul* (New York: Bantam, 1981). To me, a much more relevant question to ask today is, what is it like to be an immortal bat?

3. Reuters (February 12, 1999), story available at http://nt.excite.com/news/r/990212/03/tech-prize.

4. See http://www.organogenesis.com/docs97/tech.htm.

5. See http://www-bioc.rice.edu/Institute/Report96/page4.html.

6. See http://toad.asu.edu/rschmag/stories/101ionua.html.

7. The MIT Artificial Muscle project is at http://www.ai.mit.edu/projects/muscle/muscle.html.

8. The Artificial Muscle Research Institute of the University of New Mexico is at http://www.unm.edu/~amri/index.html.

9. Reuters (February 19, 1999), story available at http://www.wired. com:80/news/news/technology/story/18005.html.

10. W. Wayt Gibbs, "Artificial Blood Quickens: Several Short-Term Substitutes Approach Final Clinical Trials," *Scientific American* (September 1996), available at http://www.sciam.com/0996issue/ 0996techbus4.html.

11. Colin R. Johnson, "New Application Areas Addressed by Visual-Recognition Device—Vision Chip's Circuitry Modeled on Eye and Brain," *Electronic Engineering Times*, no. 971 (September 15, 1997), available at http://www.techweb.com/se/directlink.cgi?EET 19970915S0046.

12. Colin R. Johnson, "MEMS Tongue Mimics Taste Buds," *EE Times* (November 9, 1998).

13. BBC News, "World's First 'Bionic Arm' for Scot" (August 19, 1998), available at http://news.bbc.co.uk:80/hi/english/health/newsid_ 154000/154545.stm.

14. BBC News, "Deaf Man in 'Bionic' Ears Breakthrough" (September 6, 1998), available at http://news.bbc.co.uk:80/hi/english/health/news id_165000/165596.stm.

15. The press release can be found at http://www.emory.edu/WHSC/ HSNEWS/releases/feb99/022399brain.html.

16. See http://www.newscientist.com/ns/981003/editorial.html.

17. A press release from the Fraunhofer Institute for Solar Energy Systems in Germany is at http://www.ise.fhg.de/Press_Info/PI298.html.

18. A detailed technical paper by the German researchers who built the robot is available at http://www-i5.informatik.rwth-aachen.de/ gerhard/abstracts/aaai98.html.

19. Keith L. Doty and Ronald E. Van Aken, "Swarm Robot Materials Handling Paradigm for a Manufacturing Workcell," paper presented at the Institute of Electrical and Electronics Engineers (IEEE) International Conference on Robotics and Automation, Atlanta, Georgia (May 2–6, 1993). Abstract available at http://www. mil.ufl.edu/publications/abstracts/swarm.txt.

20. The relevant Johns Hopkins University Web site is at http://cae sar.me.jhu.edu/metamorphic.html.

21. Keith L. Doty and Akram Bou-Ghannam, "Controlled Situated Agent Behaviors with Perception and Cognition," undated paper (copy in author's possession). Believed to have been delivered at a meeting of the American Association for Artificial Intelligence (AAAI). Visit the AAAI Web site at http://www.aaai.org.

22. The mimeomorphic/polimorphic categorization is from sociologists H. Collins and M. Kusch, *The Shape of Actions: What Humans and Machines Can Do* (Cambridge, MA: MIT Press, 1998).

23. Read all about Cog at http://www.ai.mit.edu/projects/cog/.

CHAPTER 7

PREPARING
FOR THE FUTURE

What would happen to the health care industry if, tomorrow, the news reported genuine cures for cancer, diabetes, Parkinson's, Alzheimer's, and AIDS? When penicillin put paid (by and large) to tuberculosis, it certainly did not finish the health care industry. But it seems reasonable to assume that the number of careers in researching and diagnosing TB and caring for its victims dwindled rapidly, while the number of new careers in the management of other diseases expanded. When it takes decades between such major breakthroughs as penicillin and the polio antivirus, the health care system and its workers have time to adapt, but when dozens of breakthroughs occur annually, monthly, and even daily, adapting becomes a problem.

All the signs point to a strong likelihood that today's major diseases will succumb rapidly to the onslaught of technologies ranged against them, to the point that by the year 2030 there will be none left and that therefore those organizations and professionals that specialize in managing specific diseases and conditions (including the condition of old age) will have to be prepared for change.

Are they, and can they? Before turning the debate over to my esteemed colleagues in part 2, I will address these questions after first presenting some of the astonishing and career-threatening implications of the accelerating trends I have described in part 1.

IMPLICATIONS

Steve Heimoff, writing in *Healthcare Forum Journal* in 1998, thinks health care professionals view replacing the paper medical record as the "killer app[lication]" of the computer in medicine, and he properly notes its more advanced role as a decision support tool for caregivers. Heimoff also makes reference to "fears that computers could undermine the doctor-patient (or nurse-patient) relationship."[1]

But drawing on the key assumption that Moore's and Metcalfe's laws will continue to accelerate the development of health care–related technologies, we have arrived at a much more startling scenario, one in which the term *killer app* takes on an eery, if not downright chilling, dimension when it means the replacement of human doctors, nurses, and administrators by cyborgs and androids.

To some this will indeed seem a horrifying scenario; others will scoff at the outlandishness of it all. One physician administrator quoted in a sidebar to Heimoff's article argued that it will take from five to ten years just to get his hospital records computerized. I would argue that a mainstream medical institution lacking computerized records in five years will be an oxymoron. It will not exist; at least, not as a mainstream medical institution.

Others, however, may see a message of hope in the new bionic medium telling us that the time and the capabilities are almost upon us to explore new frontiers in inner and outer space with ageless, re-engineered bodies and augmented brains and with intelligent android companions.

An exhaustive list of implications is beyond my limited intellect and meager prophetic powers. Indeed, one of my hoped-for results from publishing this book is that others will be stimulated to contribute their thoughts—as my fellow authors have already done in part 2 of this volume. The issues are too deep and too broad for any one book even to pose all the questions let alone provide all the answers. But following are some of the implications:

- The tradition of cradle-to-grave care administered by the hometown family physician is being squeezed by the database and the smart card, which will retain more memory of the history of a patient than the family doctor can, and by telemedicine, which will enable a family in Peoria to choose a physician in Peking.

- Patients will increasingly manage their own health care and treatment, occasionally stopping by the local automated clinic, visiting a virtual clinic, or receiving a visit from a traveling robodoc equipped with all the sensors, scanners, and noninvasive surgical tools needed to examine and, if necessary, diagnose and treat the patient. The patient will wave a smart card at a card-reader, which will then arrange over the Internet for payment of the impending transaction and set the multidimensional body scan in motion, finally giving the patient a readout of its findings and recommendations (and storing them on the patient's card). If there are anomalies, the robodoc may administer manipulative or noninvasive treatment and dispense medications on the spot.
- Robodoc will have instantaneous access over a wireless Internet link to epidemiological and clinical data for comparison of the patient's symptoms, prognosis, diagnosis, and treatment options. Epidemiological and clinical data gathered from the patient will be added to the global database and instantly become integrated into an ongoing, real-time analysis of the state of human health.
- Health alerts will be automatically sent over the Internet to researchers, health policymakers, and at risk individuals.
- Over the next 30 years, individuals in the profession will at first find in technology an important aide. But the aides will eventually grow sophisticated enough to replace the human. The careers to be made in the interim are careers in biotechnology—designing, building, and managing biotech machines—until they become capable of designing, building, and managing themselves.
- With deskilling comes the imperative for reskilling, and that, coupled with the shortening half-life of medical knowledge, is why continuing medical education will assume an ever greater role in the profession.
- The practice of medicine will increasingly become characterized as high tech, low touch; and there will be astounding break-throughs in patient care and treatment. Entire medical and med-ically related careers will be eliminated, but there will also be better medicine and better health.

However startling such implications appear, they must be accepted as possible on the grounds of (1) fact and (2) reasonable assumption.

The facts are that all the technological developments discussed herein have been demonstrated, not merely conceptualized, and that acceleration in the rate of change in the computer and network technologies driving those technologies is so far obeying Moore's and Metcalfe's laws and shows no sign of a slowdown. The reasonable assumption is that this acceleration will continue, *ceteris paribus* (other things being equal), for at least the next 30 years.

Nevertheless, to abide by the rules of forecasting we should specify and consider all possible alternative scenarios. But this, too, is beyond the scope of this book, which seeks rather to present a case for the need for an exhaustive futures study. However, we can consider at least one alternative scenario by, first, relaxing the key assumption of Moore's law and, second, assuming that external factors will prevent *ceteris paribus* from holding, or both.

Relaxing the assumption by reducing Moore's annual doubling to, say, cinquennial doubling would still leave us in 30 years with thinking computers serving more as working partners than as tools we use to get work done. There would be six doublings in the power of all the technologies—a progression making it reasonable to infer, for example, that computers will be ubiquitous in offices as automated secretaries, performing filing tasks, processing bills, managing patient records, and maintaining appointment calendars and complex schedules. They will also at a minimum become surgeon assistants and perform low-level nursing and janitorial tasks.

External factors affecting the scenario would include, for example, the effect of increasing automation on the global economy. If conditions are adversely affected due to massive layoffs and resultant unemployment, lower consumption, and social unrest, then the operation of Moore's law could be stopped in its tracks or at least be considerably restricted. On the other hand, the economy could be stimulated by the technology trends I have described, producing goods, food, and services for all at low cost through robot assistants or reengineered bodies and brains, and economic growth could be nurtured and protected by enlightened (and accelerated) government and industrial leadership creating policies to mitigate the unwanted social effects of change.[2]

The fundamental message of the medium of technology has always been deskilling and the replacement of humans by machines. It has happened on the farm and in the factory and is happening in the office and lab. It is clear the trend is accelerating. The only question is how fast it is accelerating—at the pace of Moore's law or something less. The Luddites were right; only their behavior and their assessment of the pace of change were wrong. The lab technician supporting his or her family by looking through the microscope at cervical tissue cells is already being nudged aside by PAPNET, and there's lots more where that came from. The janitor is under threat from the LIDAR-equipped roaming vacuum cleaner, able to sniff out and eliminate bacteria from the hospital. Robot assistants, not the nurse's aide, will transfer patient from gurney to bed—until universal assemblers can transform the gurney into a fully equipped hospital bed under the patient's very posterior.

On the bright side, deskilling has always led to reskilling. Few Americans can ride a horse any more, but all can drive a car. Few farmers know how to thresh and flail their wheat manually, but most farmers can operate a combine harvester. Even our nuclear physicists are (blessedly) losing their memory of how to make nuclear weapons, and the key U.S. nuclear weapons laboratories are putting their physicists and mathematicians to work on solving other complex puzzles such as city traffic flows.[3]

But the people who lived through these transitions had the benefit of decades in which to convert their stables into garages and their nukes to plowshares. In contrast, a giant among U.S. stockbrokerage firms, Merrill Lynch, saw its dominance in the market fade after only about three years of competition on the new medium of the Web from the upstart Charles Schwab. At the end of 1998, Schwab overtook Merrill's market capitalization to become the leading brokerage house in America.

Major pharmacy chains may have even less time to adapt. Drugstore.com, PlanetRx.com, and Soma.com all recently began selling prescription and nonprescription drugs over the Internet. According to a Reuters newswire, the online market for drugs, vitamins, personal care, and cosmetics is estimated at $165 billion—which can be subtracted from the earnings of traditional pharmacies.[4] A message about the Internet that has been obvious for a decade is that it knows no boundaries—geopolitical or regulatory. It is amazing that people should be astonished by the availability of Viagra (not all of it genuine) over the Internet without prescription from foreign countries with nothing but hopelessly outnumbered Customs checks to stem the rising tide.

How could they let this happen? By failing to predict, and adapt to, change.

ADAPTING TO CHANGE

Remember that computers drive technology development, and technology feeds back to drive computer development in a recursive, exponentially accelerating process. I claimed in chapter 1 that few people appear to have grasped the full significance of this because the rise in the acceleration curve has so far been shallow enough and our individual minds and collective cultures have been adaptive enough that we have had just enough time to adjust to the changes wrought by the introduction of new technologies but not enough time to consider their full implications.

Does this mean that technology must slow down to a pace we can assimilate? Or does it mean that we—as individuals and organizations—must learn to assimilate and adapt to change faster? The young Charles Schwab (the individual and the organization) assimilated the implications of the Web for online trading much faster than competitors. (In the following paragraphs, what I say about the individual can easily be applied to the organization.)

The younger we are, the faster our brains adapt to new things. They have to. The mind of an infant has to cope with an avalanche of new sensory impressions, from mother's touch to the blueness of sky to the sweets and sours of food. Within the brief period of childhood and adolescence, the mind has to cope with language, social mores and institutions (family, school, perhaps church), and absorbtion of a substantial slice of the sum total of human knowledge and experience.

The great strength of the young mind is its ability to absorb cognitive shock and adapt quickly. The neurobiological basis for this capacity is now beginning to be understood. The young brain is highly plastic; that is, moldable. Biological evolution leaves the newborn brain's neural network of connections unfinished and hands over to cultural evolution the job of literally tying the loose ends together. Older brains are less plastic. There goes old Mr. Smith, set in his ways, and his old dog, unable to learn new tricks.

It is not surprising, then, that a six-year-old can become comfortable with a computer in minutes, as is well known to many a modern middle-class parent. This was turned to marketing account by Compaq, which in 1997 featured a six-year-old setting up a Presario computer and using it right out of the box. Some 60-year-old distinguished physicians will never become comfortable with one even after having been exposed to it for 20 years. With effort, anyone can adapt, but being set in one's ways is not conducive to making the effort.

Anyone can adapt because no one becomes totally rigid even if seeming to. Every brain, no matter how old, retains some measure of plasticity to cope with life changes. The brain's neural net retains the ability to reconfigure or rewire itself to some degree. If we go blind, we quickly grow better at detecting and interpreting sounds and smells—a result of the brain's rewiring its circuits to reinforce our auditory and olfactory capabilities.

Besides developmental, sensory, and injury-induced plasticity, there is a fourth type: plasticity of learning and memory, which occurs when we alter our behavior based on new cognitive information.[5] Because our present focus is on the implications of the accelerating development of computers and technology and the resulting avalanche of cognitive surprise (if not shock), it is this kind of plasticity that is most relevant in the present context. The question is: Are we plastic enough to continue absorbing an exponential increase in changes wrought by computers and technology?

One answer might be that it doesn't matter; that technology can only grow in line with our ability to absorb it so that when we reach the limit of our absorptive capability—of our plasticity of learning and memory—technology too will reach the limit of growth. This argument is based on the assumption that technology does not grow unless and until we are ready for it to grow; that we drive the vehicle of technology and could stop it at any time to alight and smell the roses. But as we saw in chapter 1, which addressed the momentum of the vehicle, that assumption may soon become untenable—a forlorn hope, if it is not already so.

The alternative answer is that we are indeed plastic enough to take whatever is thrown at us. Our brains may be designed so as to have an infinite capacity for absorption. We don't really know the brain's capacity for thought, though fair estimates have been made of its raw processing power and memory capacity vis-à-vis computers. It is noticeable that the age at which we become set in our ways has been steadily pushed back. In many countries, childhood and adolescence are very short, with children 13 or 14 years of age considered to be adults. But in Europe and the United States, many people remain immature through college and ages 20 to 25. This betokens the possibility that brain plasticity is being pushed further out by cultural evolution, and who is to say at what point this process might end? If it can be pushed from age 13 to age 25, why not to age 50, or 80? The growing prevalence of adult education and lifelong learning, the dispatch of a 70-year-old U.S. senator to space, and, in the professions, continuing professional education are a response to the acceleration in new knowledge and a factor forcing plasticity to extend further out.

But there is a third possible answer; namely, that technology will make up for any lack of plasticity. To own and operate one of the earliest automobiles, you had to become a mechanic. To operate an early computer, you had to become a computer scientist. But today millions drive cars and run computers with no idea of how they work. The day might come when all of us can visit space without being trained as astronauts or perform brain surgery as easily as cooking up a meal in the microwave. *Star Trek: The Next Generation*'s Dr. Crusher seems to have the easiest job on the *Enterprise*. With a wave of her magic medical wand, she diagnoses and treats her patients in one fell, noninvasive swoop. Heck, I could do that. So, for that matter, could Rover, my pet dogbot.

In short, one way or another we will keep pace with technological developments, and the acceleration described in this book will not slow down just because some of us might want it to.

Whether you like these implications or not, if you accept that they have some credibility, then you are best advised to strive to anticipate them if you are to have any hope of influencing them or ameliorating their effects on your organization, your life, your career, and your profession.

But how? It would be nice to think that all one needs to do is to read this book, but not even I could maintain that conceit for very long. The issues are, as I said before, too deep and too broad for any one mind to grasp in their entirety. They are also too nebulous to be amenable to traditional scientific and social-scientific research methods. Neural nets and other state-of-the-art research tools, which have already begun to make substantial and successful inroads into such nebulous areas as weather and economic forecasting, might be applied, but they won't reach their full potential until the 30 years we want to predict is up.

For the individual health care organization the answer is twofold. First, appoint an executive or consultant to keep the organization informed of technological developments that might affect it. Some organizations are already doing this: One of the contributors to this book, Brian Peters, is responsible for health care futures at the Michigan Health & Hospital Association; and another contributor, Donald Crandall, cannot avoid looking to the future in his capacity as vice president for clinical informatics at Mercy Health Services.

Second, I echo the suggestion of Stuart Davidson that health care organizations hold technology reviews at least once every 18 months. Eighteen months, you will recall, is all it takes (on average) for the computer chips on which the future of health care rests to double in power. It will give the organization the chance to consider which of the technologies they have invested in, or intend to invest in, are what Davidson calls "half-way" technologies[6] (for example, the iron lung), and which ones are likely to have staying power and can be depreciated/ amortized, written off against taxes, or resold to third world, veterinary, and other organizations that may not be able to afford the latest technology by the time the next generation of replacement technology appears.

These are steps that need to be taken now. In 10 years' time, the trend toward DIY health care and inexpensive health care technologies for home use could mean that health care consumers themselves will be conducting such reviews, in the informal way in which people today consider the pros and cons of replacing their PC every couple of years. One of the first questions many now ask is: How long will it be before the new machine I buy will be obsolete, unable to handle the increasingly power-hungry programs I suspect I am going to want to use?

Neither the individual "chief futures officer," if I may coin a term, nor the 18-month review panel have the time it takes to look very far ahead, and their employers will prefer they spend their time on the relatively short-term future. The further ahead we want to look (in any sort of valid and reliable way), the more resources we have to put into it. I believe the topic of this book is deserving of a full-blown, longitudinal futures study, funded by philanthropic and government bodies and involving every facet of the health care industry.

FUTURES STUDIES

The field of futures studies is a relatively new professional discipline, arising in the 1950s and 1960s in response to growing complexity and change.[7] Its methodologies, invented in think tanks and activist organizations, include content analysis, scenarios, cross-impact analysis, and adaptations of the old Delphi brainstorming method.

The field is different from but connected to traditional forecasting and planning disciplines. It typically looks forward 10 to 50 years, whereas economists and market researchers typically look out one to three years. It focuses on systemic, transformational change as opposed to incremental changes from existing trends. It forecasts multiple *alternative, possible,* and *preferable* future scenarios rather than single predictions. And it uses qualitative and indirect/derivative as well as direct quantitative methodologies (particularly demographic projections from statistical data), where traditional forecasting tends to rely on direct quantitative tools.

A scenario is an illustrative outline or a synopsis of coming events. It should not pretend to represent the full spectrum of possibilities. A scenario has a low probability of resembling accurately the actual future course of history, but—and this is the key—if properly conducted, it will have a reasonable possibility of pointing in the direction of truth and serving as a yardstick against which to measure specific predictions and assumptions.

Forecasting by means of scenario building is more like "mapping a cone of uncertainty" (Paul Saffo, Institute for the Future[8]) than predicting a specific and certain outcome. It is a process of mapping ignorance. A forecast can be designed to reduce uncertainty by allowing its recipient not merely to lie in wait for a predicted outcome and then react to it but to take action to influence the outcome ahead of time.

I am grateful to Pat Grauer of the Michigan State University College of Osteopathic Medicine for pointing out to me that the process may also have a built-in Hawthorne Effect, meaning that the very act of studying the future may produce a better one, in the same way that workers at Western Electric's Hawthorne plant worked more productively no matter what changes in working conditions—within limits, good or bad—were imposed on them. They did so, the researchers concluded, simply because they were happy someone was paying attention to them.

One futurist (Lawrence Wilkinson, Global Business Network[9]) has suggested that although the scenario process is best applied to specific problems—"Should I build a new plant, or buy a company, or get out of a business?"—it is nevertheless important also to identify and forecast the social, political, economic, and technical context surrounding the problem. This latter is what analytical writers like Alvin Toffler (*Future Shock*) and John Naisbitt (*Megatrends*) do so well, and they do it using a process called *content analysis*. Basically, they employ teams of documentary researchers to read through hundreds of newspapers and magazines over a long period of time, culling and collating factual information (not editorial opinion) about social, economic, and other issues.

Armed with a few years' worth of such collated information, it is not difficult to write a book like *Megatrends*. I know, because I did something similar in a former incarnation as a China watcher for the British and Hong Kong governments, and also on a smaller scale for Ameritech in 1988. I also used the technique in building a business plan in 1989–1990 for an online service and in writing this book. In the first three cases, my 10- to 20-year predictions have turned out to be pretty accurate. The company I founded remains afloat in the turbulent waters of the Internet business, Ameritech has handled the uncertainties of the past decade in some respects better than the other Baby Bells, and Britain and China settled the Hong Kong question amicably. This is not to boast; my contributions were miniscule in the overall scheme of things, but it does illustrate that content analysis works.

For example, in South Africa the Montfleur project, designed to secure the country's future in a postapartheid world, brought together such unlikely bedfellows as the "one settler, one bullet" Pan-African Congress with rabid white supremacists as well as with the moderate African National Congress, the Incata movement, the chamber of commerce, the government, and unions. Together they forecast a set of scenarios, published in the South African press, that convinced enough people that the current path spelled doom for all and that a different future could be good for all.[10] A key product of this work was the mandated Truth and Reconciliation Commission, charged with uncovering the truth about apartheid-era abuses, reconciling the country's divided races, granting amnesty to those who confessed political crimes in full, and paying compensation to victims.

There are writers, including not just science fiction writers but academics, who predict war between humans and intelligent machines in 30 years. In *The March of the Machines*, Professor Kevin Warwick paints a scenario of an aggressive race of robots ruling the world in 30 to 40 years or even sooner: "By 2025, many of us might well be under the marching orders of these little machines and their networked superiors. . . . [T]here is no feasible reason why we won't be, unless we fight back." Hugo de Garis, the "brain builder," also predicts a bloodbath between humans and what he calls "artilects," for artificial intellects.

I think these notions are nonsense, but it has taken another whole book (not yet published) to explain why, and it is neither necessary nor appropriate to go into the reasons here. I mention these examples to show: first, that intelligent people predict extraordinary developments in technology; second, that they generally agree on a 30-year time frame; and, third, that there is disagreement over the nature of the developments. Whether the next 30 years will bring a wasteland or the Promised Land is something we surely ought to try to find out.

In part 2 of this book, six professionals in the health care field—a physician, a nurse, a hospital association executive, two insurance executives, and a strategic consultant—provide rather more thoughtful and less exotic perspectives than Professors Warwick and de Garis might offer and that I offer on the impacts of future technology trends on their respective industries. They have responded to my challenge in a welcome variety of ways.

Dr. Don Crandall brings a lifetime of distinguished service to the medical community and his technology-savvy physician's knowledge and perspective to bear in describing trends in clinical decision making. He foresees, as I do, a future in which technology empowers the patient to be an equal partner with the physician in diagnosis and treatment.

Nurse and writer Meg Campbell offers a bold and highly readable description of a day in the life of a critical care unit in the year 2030 compared with a CCU today. Like her fellow contributors, Meg is less aggressive about the future than I am, but she sees—as do I—a loss of nursing jobs to computers and robots but at the same time a higher-level role for the nurses who remain.

Brian Peters also sees a greater role for patients and a dramatic aging of the population. These views come not from a crystal ball but from his observations of today's trends. He presents evidence that the aging of America has already dramatically affected the American hospital. He also makes the telling remark that "technology development outpaces the wisdom to deal with it," though he foresees the pace as being slow enough to give the hospital time to redefine itself as being in the business of health, not just inpatient care. My own opinion is that hospitals will very soon need to redefine themselves again as being in the business of superhealth.

Marianne Udow and Kevin Seitz also take a "more modest and cautious" view of the future. In their everyday world as health insurers, "success with automation is still measured largely by a payer's percentage of electronically transmitted claims," and they not unreasonably point to the danger of succumbing to technology hype when making short-term business decisions. They too acknowledge the trend to consumerism and recognize that their industry will therefore need to provide better customer service. They make the important point that the trend to consumerism in health care has political implications, at least in the United States, where special interests will find their power to influence legislation eroded by the growing power of consumers.

Craig Ruff eloquently—though purely incidentally—makes the case for reading this book, at least for reading key books and articles dealing with science and technology, some of which he describes. Craig's message is that as a leader in health care, you need to know that technology is empowering, and you therefore need to know something about technology; and that as a follower, you need also to know something about technology in order to be able to hold your leaders to account for their use, nonuse, misuse, or abuse of it.

References and Notes

1. Steve Heimoff, "The Forces That Impact Healthcare—Technology," *Healthcare Forum Journal* (January/February, 1998): 14–19.

2. Some economists argue that to survive, capitalism necessarily depends on technological infrastructure growth and ever higher spending, analogous to the industrial age when capitalism depended on huge infrastructure projects such as dams and railroads (but then, it seems to me, so did socialism). See, for example, a short Listserv discussion at http://www.pix.org/pof/econ_moore.htm.

3. Donald MacKenzie presents a cogent thesis that with the passage of the old guard of nuclear physicists who had practical hands-on experience of the enormously complex process of building and testing real bombs as opposed to supercomputer simulations of them, the United States may soon be hard-pressed to make any more. His thesis explains why Iraq, after years of effort and enormous expense, has not succeeded in making a bomb. See Donald MacKenzie, *Knowing Machines: Essays on Technical Change* (Cambridge, MA: MIT Press, 1996).

4. Reuters (February 24, 1999), story available at http://www.wired. com/news/news/email/explode-infobeat/business/story/18101.html.

5. My categorization of plasticities differs slightly from the current standard categorization. Vanderbilt University categorizes them as "[first,] when the immature brain first begins to process sensory information (developmental plasticity); second, when changes in the body, like a problem with eyesight, alter the balance of sensory activity received by the brain (activity-dependent plasticity); third, when we alter our behavior based on new sensory information (plasticity of learning and memory); and fourth, following damage to the brain (injury-induced plasticity)." See http://www.vander bilt.edu/kennedy/brainpl.html.

6. Stuart Davidson, "Technological Cancer: Its Causes and Treatment," *Healthcare Forum Journal* (March/April, 1995).

7. Parts of this description of the field of futures studies are paraphrased from the program for the MS course in Studies of the Future at the University of Houston-Clear Lake. See http://www.cl. uh.edu/futureweb/program.html.

8. For more information about future studies in general and the Institute for the Future in particular, visit http://www.iftf.org/.

9. The Global Business Network can be found at http://www.gbn.org/ home.html.

10. GBN's Lawrence Wilkinson discussed the Montfleur project in an October 25, 1995, chat session on *HotWired*. The session transcript can be read at http://www.hotwired.com/talk/club/special/tran scripts/wilkinson.html.

PROFESSIONAL PERSPECTIVES

CHAPTER 8

THE PROCESS OF THE HEALTH CARE ENCOUNTER

Donald K. Crandall, MD, FACS

D uring the past 25 years we have witnessed seemingly independent but parallel advancements in the areas of computer science, communication technology, and biotechnology. Computer performance has increased at the accelerated rates demonstrated by Moore's law. Communication technology is now satellite based, worldwide, and with high bandwidths for improved transmission of high-resolution images and rapid communication. The Human Genome Project and other biotechnical advances are rapidly changing our understanding of the disease process and treatment options. These seemingly independent advances are rapidly converging, the lines between the different disciplines are disappearing, and a major area of this fusion of technologies will be applied in the health care encounter of the future.

THE CLINICAL DECISION-MAKING PROCESS

With advances in computerization, communication, and biotechnology and increasing economic and political pressures, the entire clinical decision-making process is being challenged. Significant variation in the observations, perceptions, and interpretation of data have resulted in significant variation in the utilization and quality of health care in this country. David Eddy, MD, has stated that "the solution is not to remove the decision-making power from physicians, but to improve the capacity of the physicians to make better decisions."[1] To achieve this solution we need to use advances in computerization and communication to give physicians the information they need at the time and place the clinical decision is made.

The following are four approaches to clinical decision making as outlined by Eddy.[2]

1. *Global subjective judgment,* where the decision maker performs all tasks subjectively based on personal or global experience, is currently the usual approach to clinical decision making.

2. The *evidence-based approach* explicitly and systematically describes all pertinent evidence and rates the strengths of this evidence. Several consensus panel reports have recently been published in an effort to expand this evidence-based approach.

3. The *outcomes-based approach* not only considers the available evidence but also uses the important outcomes of the health intervention and alternative interventions in the decision-making process.

4. The *preference-based approach* includes an assessment of the patient's preferences for the outcomes.

Global subjective judgment has been the time-honored approach to medical decision making and is still used to a great extent. Nevertheless, significant headway has been made recently in the utilization of evidence-based medicine. It is becoming part of the curriculum in medical schools and residency programs, and Web sites devoted to science and teaching of evidence-based medicine are available. The rapid expansion of clinical trials, computer analysis of results, and widespread communication will result in the expansion of evidence-based medicine. Ultimately, this approach will be incorporated into practice policies or clinical guidelines and interfaced with specific patient data to facilitate the clinical decision-making process.

The outcomes-based approach to clinical decision making will be expanded as worldwide studies are added to the current database and data-mining tools are developed to extract, analyze, communicate, and incorporate the knowledge of outcomes.

The preference-based approach will require patients' understanding of the different outcomes to different therapies. Web-based information has already resulted in a more knowledgeable public and will make future attempts by insurers to limit certain treatments more difficult. On the other hand, ineffective treatments and bad outcomes should be eliminated by this increase in knowledge, resulting in higher-quality, more consistent health care.

COMPUTERIZATION OF THE HEALTH CARE ENCOUNTER

There are increasing demands by the government, employers, and patients to improve the quality, consistency, and value of health care in this country. The approach to date has been primarily focused on fine-tuning the system as we know it, making small changes at the periphery. This has resulted in minimal improvements in the quality, consistency, and value of health care. In order to achieve the changes needed for the future, more substantive changes in the way we deliver health care are needed.

Computerized Health Information Systems

Merely tampering with the system by altering the financing mechanism for payment for service has not resulted, and will not result, in the changes needed to meet the demands on the system in the coming years. Commitment to the computerization of the financial system currently lacks emphasis on the clinical side of health care. We will not meet our quality and cost objectives until the computerization of the design, manufacturing, and delivery of the health care service is addressed. This will happen only with the implementation of an integrated computerized health information system that will track patient activity and outcomes across the continuum of care. The extreme fragmentation of the health care delivery system has led to a fragmentation of the available data as well. The problem is a lack of timely, reliable, relevant, and usable data. Deriving more value from existing data and converting data into information and knowledge will be the major objectives for health information systems in the near future.

There are integrated computerized hospital information systems in use today that interface with the patient-physician encounter, but these are limited in scope and use.[3] To be successful in the future, a health system will need to develop an electronic patient information system that will allow access to sequential episodic patient treatment, outcome, and satisfaction information over a period of time in a longitudinal patient record.[4] Currently, there are many computer applications in use that address only the components of a patient's health care encounter. To meet the needs of true integration of care we need to simplify, integrate, and automate the collection, analysis, and distribution of medical information to be used at the patient-specific decision level.

Historically, computerization in the health care industry has developed one proprietary application at a time. The applications were usually hospital based, task oriented, and with closed architecture. As a result, hospitals have many different computer systems, but communication between systems, integration of data, and conversion of the data to useful information are difficult and expensive. The information system of the future will have open architecture, be integrated and patient centered, with greater focus on quality and outcome measures. Standards in data definition will be expanded so data can be compared across providers and systems to identify best-practice methods. Automatic data entry at point of service in a digital format for easy storage and transmission will be expanded. Patient demographic information, clinical data, laboratory results, pharmaceutical systems, and patient preferences will be integrated and used in the clinical decision-making process at the point of service. Web site technology will be used to allow easy access to the data warehouses from remote sites. This will be used to create a virtual network of providers to expand the patient base of the health care system.

Clinical Data Repositories. Data warehouses are useful for tracking progress, either for marketing, profiling, or outcomes analysis, whereas clinical data repositories are actually used in the process of patient care. Data warehousing is a way to bring together data from a wide range of disciplines to enable new analysis. It is an information systems building block that will eventually become a cornerstone of enterprise information systems architectures.[5] Clinical data repositories are systems that store and retrieve clinical data electronically. These systems provide the foundation technology for electronic records. In a recent survey, almost 60 percent of health care providers responding stated they were implementing or planning to implement clinical data repositories.[6]

Electronic Medical Records. More than 97 percent of health care encounters occur outside the hospital setting, requiring data to be captured at the point of care. Currently, the electronic medical record (EMR) is being incorporated into many physician practices. Several issues need to be addressed to expand the usefulness of the EMR.

Interfacing the system to other sources of patient data will need to be expanded so that information will be captured once and then shared across the system. New data-capture and data-entry devices will be incorporated into the system to make data collection easier and more accurate. Care processes, outcomes, and patient satisfaction will be automatically monitored. Neural networks will be used to analyze large numbers of previous health encounters to aid in more rapid diagnosis based on the available clinical data. Treatment processes will be identified that result in the best outcomes and satisfaction. These data, along with evidence-based practice protocols developed from extensive data mining of worldwide clinical studies, will be integrated in the computer. These data will be coupled with the specific genetic makeup of the patient to assess patient-specific risks and determine the most effective diagnostic and treatment plan. As best practices are more easily identified and shared among providers of health services, we will see a significant reduction in variation and greater standardization and efficiency in the delivery of health services.

With the advent of individual genetic makeup and patient risk profiling, access to a patient's record becomes a significant concern. Physicians are testing a new record system that allows patients to carry their medical information around with them on a computer chip attached to a wristband. This new system documents a patient's progress from preoperative testing through anesthesia and recovery.[7] Smart cards will be used as patient records to allow point-of-service data entry and retrieval. Security will be enhanced by thumb print or retinal identification. As microtechnology advances, one's entire health record will be kept on a computer chip imbedded in the person.

Patient Confidentiality and Confidence

One of the first steps in developing a networked health enterprise is to develop a common patient identifier or Enterprise Master Person Index (EMPI) to link information about a patient from several data sources across the continuum of care. The creation of a common patient identifier immediately raises concerns about confidentiality and data protection.

Data protection has two aspects: security and integrity.[8] Security means data must be protected against unauthorized access; integrity means that data must be valid and accessible.

Security Issues. The Health Insurance Portability and Accountability Act (HIPAA) of 1996 mandated the unique patient identifier, but the American Medical Association (AMA) has said it cannot support its use until medical necessity and security issues are resolved.[9] The concerns of patients about the confidentially of medical records were highlighted in a recent report from the AMA board of trustees showing that increasing electronic data collection and transmission have increased patient fears and decreased their trust in our health care system.[10] HIPAA (PL 104–191) highlighted the necessity for statutory guidance on the issue of medical record confidentiality. Congress has until August 1999 to pass national legislation that addresses the issues of rights of individuals who are the subject of identifiable health information, the procedure for exercising those rights, and how disclosure is authorized.[11] It was stated in recent roundtable discussions among health care leaders that "inappropriate treatment due to bad information is a greater risk than the risk of transferring information inappropriately."[12] However, new AMA guidelines go beyond current legislative or regulatory proposals and state that a patient's right to privacy supersedes all other institutional and individual needs for medical information. The AMA believes patient consent is a firewall protecting medical information and doesn't want technological efficiency or administrative simplification to supersede the right of patients to privacy.[13]

Integrity Issues. Information integrity is a concern to both the public and the provider of health care. When clinical data are used for clinical decision making, identifying best practices, and comparing outcomes and cost, it is paramount that the information be valid. Before physicians will embrace the use of computer-generated data in the clinical decision-making process, they will need to be assured of the validity of the data. There are currently systems available for data standardization, validation, verification, scrubbing, and grouping that are applied to data retrieval and storage. Widespread confidence in these systems is necessary as we move forward in the development of networked health enterprises. Until the issues surrounding patient confidentiality and confidence are resolved to the satisfaction of the public, the implementation of evolving technologies and their benefits are at risk of being significantly delayed.

EMERGING TECHNOLOGIES

Deloitte & Touche recently surveyed the health care industry to identify trends in the implementation of health management technology. They categorized the trends as "information access enabling" or "productivity enabling" technologies. The most frequent technologies in information access enabling were in multimedia, handheld computers, data warehouse/decision support, and the Internet. The productivity enabling technologies were expert systems/neural networks, automated call centers, voice recognition, object-oriented technology, work flow management, groupware, and image/document management.[14] Many of these technologies, as well as other emerging technologies, are rapidly changing the process of the health care encounter. The closer look at some of these technologies that this book provides will give insight into its future.

Telemedicine

The concept of telemedicine typically refers to the use of telecommunications technologies to facilitate health care delivery. Many telemedicine applications are already in place and providing the benefits of improved access to expertise and information, lower service costs, reduced isolation, and improved quality of care. Networks linking multiple hospitals, research centers, and remote health clinics allow isolated rural communities access to specialty consultation and state-of-the-art treatment options. Physician-to-hospital linkage is in place to transmit patient information, laboratory results, electrocardiograms, and radiologic images to a clinical workstation that can be accessed at the patient encounter and from remote sites. Through e-mail technology, the results can be forwarded to patients or other health care providers.

Videoconferencing and personal computer teleconferencing when patient and provider are physically separated are the latest trends in telemedicine. Video links are being used for patient diagnostic and monitoring encounters. Home-care telemedicine provides a process of interacting with a patient remotely.

Most basic video systems include a small video camera and screen for transmitting and displaying video signals. The system can be augmented with the addition of an otoscope, a blood glucose meter, blood pressure cuff, or cardiogram to support a specific diagnosis.[15] Peak flow meters to measure air flow in asthmatics have been connected to home computers, the results transmitted to a physician, and adjustments made to the treatment plan based on the new data. With the development of diagnosis-specific treatment algorithms, the computer system will be able to make the necessary changes to a treatment plan.

Current videoconferencing can be transmitted over standard analog telephone lines. Telemedicine is primarily a monitoring device today. As transmission speeds increase with advances in telecommunication technologies, more real-time interactive health care encounters will take place. With the development of microtechnology-based sensors and high-bandwidth data links, the health care encounter will move into the arena of virtual reality. These online consultations are changing the way medicine is practiced, challenging the expectations of patients, and raising a number of professional and ethical issues along the way.[16]

Web-Based Medicine

In a recent survey by the Healthcare Information and Management Systems Society (HIMSS) and Hewlett Packard (HP) Leadership, it was found that 87 percent of health care organizations are currently using the Internet.[17] Web-based medicine will see rapid expansion as the public's use of the Internet for both information and commerce increases.

The major use of the Internet in the health care industry is for information transfer. Hospitals are connecting their physicians to a wealth of information through Web-based systems. Columbia-Presbyterian has developed a program that electronically reminds physicians and their patients about necessary immunizations.[18] However, a survey by Deloitte & Touche found that although 80 percent of hospitals use the Internet, only 16 percent use it to give information directly to patients. The Internet will allow a significant shift in educational techniques from "broadcast to interactive medicine."[19]

Both patients and physicians are referring to the Internet for disease-specific information. A recent survey by CDB Research & Consulting Inc. of New York shows nearly half of all physicians (46 percent) access medical information on the Internet, and that 94 percent of these physicians said it improves their ability to provide health care.[20] Patients are approaching their health care encounter armed with medical information they have found via the Internet. Significantly, 77 percent of patients prefer to get online health information directly from their own physicians, but only 10 percent of doctors have a Web page.[21]

Physicians' use of the Internet ranges from not at all to wired and loving it. Patient education and e-mail continue to be widely used applications, and most practices have recognized the marketing potential of posting a Web site. But while some physicians are breaking new ground with patient and provider interactivity via the Web, others continue to take a wait-and-see approach. Patient education, patient e-mail, and marketing a practice online are current uses of Web-based medicine.[22] The Internet is a growing way for health plans to deliver a value-added service by communicating with the public about provider data, health education, and health plan benefits.[23]

Web-based consultations are a natural extension of telemedicine, and there will be a significant increase in patient-initiated consultations, creating opportunities for the expansion of a virtual health network. Hospitals will use Internet commerce to provide customers with information about their people, products, services, and quality. Web technology will improve customer service, lower operating costs, personalize service, and integrate existing systems. Internet technology can be applied to a clinical trials database, making it easier to match patients with specific clinical trials, which will increases the odds of patient participation and decease the drudgery for physicians.[24]

"When it comes to increasing drug prescribing via the Internet, there's a cyberclash brewing. Legal experts and medical ethicists are butting heads with technology advocates and business opportunists."[25] Recent advances in sexual performance drugs have created an instant Internet market for drugs. The legal and ethical implication of prescribing over the Internet without a traditional doctor-patient relationship will be weighed against the cost and convenience of Internet commerce.

Continuing medical education (CME), residency training, and medical student education are being conducted online. Many Internet training programs, both accredited and nonaccredited, are currently available online.[26] The future will bring increasing opportunities for online medical education. A wide range of course work will be offered with online faculty interaction. As communication technology improves, online monitoring and evaluation of individual knowledge and skills will be done and communicated to the public via Internet technology.

Using Web-enabling technology, Internet tools are being used to access traditional data and applications via Web servers and Web browsers. Health systems intranets are linking caregivers and patients to systemwide information. The Indianapolis Network for Patient Care uses an intranet to link many of the city's emergency departments for real-time access to patient records. Emergency department records are tracked, stored, and retrieved using Web-based technologies.[27]

Human Genome Project

In the fall of 1988, the multibillion-dollar Human Genome Research project was launched. It may prove to be the most significant scientific project of the twentieth century—our way of life is likely to be more fundamentally transformed in the next several decades than in the previous thousand years. Private commercial ventures and other governments have joined to establish their own genome project for plants, microorganisms, and numerous animal species.

The initial intent of the Human Genome Project was to map, sequence, and characterize all human chromosomes in order to facilitate more effective discovery of genes involved in disease and other biological processes. Since the initiation of the project, it has rapidly evolved from this genetic focus to encompass a much wider set of disciplines in biology. This growth has resulted in an explosion of advances in both information and technology. Genomics now encompasses large-scale sequencing of genes, comparative analysis of these sequences, gene expression analysis, positional cloning of disease susceptibility genes, and biochemical pathway discovery.[28]

There has been significant advancement in the understanding of numerous monogenetic diseases such as cystic fibrosis and Huntington's disease, where the presence of a specific gene can account for the disease. However, in Alzheimer's disease (AD), research has identified four genes involved in the genetic risk. It is clear, however, that other genetic risk factors for the common form of AD must exist, as these four factors account for only 50 percent of the total genetic risk.[29] Although genetic factors play a prominent role in AD, epidemiological and molecular genetic data suggest that there are likely multiple etiologies.[30]

Research strategies to understand the role of genetic variation in determining variation in the risk of common multifactorial diseases (such as coronary artery disease, diabetes, hypertension, and behavioral disorders) are under way. One must consider the possibility that the endpoint of the emergent property of these diseases may depend on environmental factors as well as genetic makeup, and one must evaluate the contribution of genetic and environmental factors to predict the individual variation in the risk of exhibiting the disease.[31] There is no known combination of phenotypes in an individual for which risk is totally absent or disease an absolute certainty. Biological risk factors are explained by the interaction of the effects of differences in many genes with exposures to variation in numerous environmental factors.[32]

DNA Chips

One of the major benefits of the Human Genome Project has been the advance in genetic research technology. Conventional gene-mapping techniques look at a relatively small number of genetic markers. The recent advancement in DNA chip technology makes it possible for an entire genome to be analyzed in a single step.[33] Today's DNA chips contain more than 40,000 probes. This achievement should aid efforts to map multigene traits.

Silicon microfabrication technology has made it possible to develop miniature analytical thermal cycling instruments to perform real-time fluorescence monitoring of DNA production that can be used to identify and analyze human genes and pathogenic viruses and bacteria.[34] This will lead to the ability to take a small sample of a patient's DNA and map his or her entire genetic makeup, identifying individual disease susceptibility, outlining a personal diagnostic and treatment program, and predicting what drug therapy will be effective against his or her specific illness. It will also allow rational approaches to preventive health measures.

THE BIOTECH CENTURY

In his recent book *The Biotech Century*,[35] Jeremy Rifkin describes the following technological and social forces coming together to create the matrix for the coming biotech advances:

- The ability to isolate, identify, and recombine genes
- The awarding of patents on gene, cell lines, genetically engineered tissue, organs, and organisms
- The globalization of commerce
- Mapping the human genome
- Studies on the genetic basis of human behavior
- The fusing of computational and genetic technologies
- A new cosmological narrative about evolution

Genomics and informatics will be the dominant growth industries of the early twenty-first century. The convergence of genomics and information heralds a new era of biomedical research, offering unbridled opportunities for bioentrepreneurs. A handful of global corporations, research institutions, and governments could hold patents on virtually all 100,000 genes that make up the blueprints of the human race, as well as the cells, organs, and tissues that comprise the human body.

We are in the process of building the technology platforms and infrastructures for molecular medicine. The development of information tools to annotate, archive, and analyze the vast volume and diversity of datasets that will be generated will be a key factor in research progress. Data mining in bioinformatics, cheminformatics, and population genetics will lead to the identification of new molecular targets for drug action. Research in molecular diagnostics and pharmacogenomics will lead to the identification of disease-associated molecular targets for drug discovery. Numerous molecular markers are being identified that can be used in the diagnosis, staging, and stratification of important diseases.[36] Automated mass spectrometry allows simultaneous assay of tens of thousands of analytes, which will accelerate the research process significantly. Developments in vector technology, gene delivery, and gene expression control methods are constantly driving the field forward.

Gene Therapy

Some of the initial work in gene therapy involved the introduction of specific genes in animals, which resulted in the production of monoclonal antibodies, anticlotting drugs, and human hemoglobin. We are already using genetically engineered drugs such as human insulin, erythropoietin, and plasminogen activator (tPA) for the treatment of heart disease, cancer, AIDS, and stroke. Advances are being made in the development of artificial cells, such as using a biodegradable polymer to wrap the hemoglobin molecule in a nanocapsule, resulting in a synthetic hemoglobin molecules design for short-term oxygen transport in critical situations.[37] Catalytic RNA molecules are under development that have the potential to selectively control gene expression in a highly specific way that could impact disorders involving gene expression.[38] Transgenetic plants will be developed to serve as pharmaceutical factories for the production of chemicals and drugs, and transgenetic animals will be used to produce human replacement organs.

One of the measures stemming from the Human Genome Project is an advance in gene therapy or pharmacogenomics that is being developed to address specific genetic diseases. Gene therapy is already in use in the treatment of cancer, Huntington's disease, and Parkinson's disease. Initial efforts in gene therapy have been directed at somatic therapy, where the genetic change affects the individual cells being treated.

There is currently interest in germ-line intervention where genes are transplanted into the sperm, egg, or embryonic cell and the genetic changes are passed along to future generations. With this new technology we can move into the arena of negative eugenics, which involves elimination of so-called undesirable biologic traits. The next step would be positive eugenics using selective breeding with gene manipulation to improve the characteristics of an organism or species. This allows for the reengineering of the human genetic blueprint and redefines the process of evolution. As a result, new quandaries have emerged about altering an individual's genetic heritage—ostensibly to cure diseases, but inevitably to effect more cosmetic changes in the human genome.[39] Unless the public is reassured that the requisite protections are in place to avoid the abusive uses of genetics, public concern and alarm will deflect progress, and the full benefits of genetic medicine will be delayed or, worse still, abandoned.

In the past, genetic testing concerned the next generation: decisions about an unborn child (for example, Tay-Sachs disease, cystic fibrosis, and Down's syndrome) and screening of newborns (for such conditions as phenylketonuria and sickle cell anemia). Increasingly, genetic testing now concerns the current generation—testing ourselves for susceptibility to chronic disease. There are four uncertainties with genetic testing that clinicians will have to communicate to patients: (1) the nature of the risk; (2) the generalizability of risk estimates; (3) the time at which risk information is useful; and (4) the utility of intervention. Population-based risk estimates should be obtained before acting on genetic data.[40] With the wider application of genetic testing, concerns are raised about the insurability of those individuals who are at greater risk for certain types of chronic disease. It is felt that insurance companies and health providers are the most likely to practice genetic discrimination. Companies may also plan to conduct routine genetic-screening tests of their prospective employees and dependents. This could lead to an informal genetic caste system. Highlights of AMA guidelines to safeguard patient privacy and confidentiality state that "genetic information should not be disclosed to third parties without the explicit informed consent of the patient."[41]

Drug Design

As genomics is uncovering the roots of disease, pharmacogenomics is allowing drug companies to see which compounds may work on specific disease-causing protein, indicating a very specific target for the drug to attack. Currently, just 20 to 40 percent of people respond to a given medicine. Drug company researchers believe the low response rate could be caused by normal genetic variations among people that make them more or less susceptible to the effects of a drug.

"In an unprecedented shift of resources and research, the nation's largest pharmaceutical companies are turning their focus toward the root causes of diseases and away from the development of drugs that treat only symptoms."[42] Pharmaceutical companies are concentrating on developing a new generation of drugs that strikes disease at their genetic and molecular levels. We should be able to determine each person's genetic risk factors and, based on lifestyles, we should be able to individualize their drug therapy. Faster testing and development of drugs has resulted from advances in high-throughput screening and retrieval of chemical and biological compounds. In the 1980s, companies had the capability of screening about 10,000 compounds per year. In the early 1990s that increased to over 10,000 per month.[43] Despite this rapid development of future drug therapies, significant challenges will face us in the near future.

INFECTIONS AND THE COMING PLAGUE

Infectious diseases have returned with a vengeance despite hopes in the 1960s that they would be virtually eliminated as a significant factor in social life. Infectious diseases are now the leading cause of death worldwide and the third leading cause of death in the United States. Between 1980 and 1992, infectious disease deaths increased by 58 percent; the major contributors were HIV infection and AIDS, respiratory disease (primarily pneumonia), and bloodstream infection.

A glance back in history shows the last case of smallpox documented in the United States was 1949, and in 1977 smallpox was eradicated worldwide. From 1985 through 1994 the number of reported cases of poliomyelitis decreased 84 percent, from more than 39,000 to 6,241. Diphtheria is an infectious disease that is rarely seen in the United States today. However, a breakdown of public health measures and immunization levels in the former Soviet Union has resulted in an increase in reported cases of diphtheria from 839 in 1989 to 47,802 in 1994, with 1,746 deaths.[44]

Despite historical predictions that infectious disease would wane in the United States, data show that infectious disease mortality in the United States has been increasing in recent years. Between 1980 and 1992, the death rate due to infectious diseases as the underlying cause of death increased 58 percent, from 41 to 65 deaths per 100,000 population in the United States.[45] In her book *The Coming Plague*, Laurie Garrett has detailed the factors involved with, and the risk of, the emerging diseases such as Lassa fever, Ebola, HIV, and increasing drug-resistant bacteria, viruses, and parasites.[46]

Human immunodeficiency virus (HIV) is the most significant emerging infectious pathogen of this century. Pathogens such as HIV that mutate extensively present significant challenges to effective monitoring of pathogens and to disease control. Naturally occurring mutations in HIV-1–infected patients have important implications for therapy and the outcomes of clinical studies. Mutation results in viruses resistant to as many as six PRI drugs.

Protease-sequencing chips are used to analyze amino acid changes known to contribute to drug resistance.[47] With this new sequencing chip technology, we will be able to identify drug resistance prior to initiation of treatment. Advances in computer technology and information transfer are resulting in more timely reporting and dissemination of data that are important elements of surveillance.[48]

The Postantimicrobial Era

One of the primary causes of the increase in infectious disease is the emergence of antimicrobial resistance. Antimicrobial resistance exhibits important epidemiological characteristics: inappropriate physician prescribing practices, the increasing mobility of the earth's population, and amplification of resistance by person-to-person and common-source transmission of resistant microorganisms in crowded institutional settings.

One must weigh the potential benefits of antimicrobial prophylaxis or empiric therapy in an individual patient against the cost and consequences of antimicrobial resistance at large.[49] The strategy for minimizing the impact of drug-resistant organisms focuses on (1) implementing an electronic laboratory-based surveillance (ELBS) system for reporting invasive infections and providing clinically relevant feedback to clinicians, (2) identifying risk factors and outcomes, (3) increasing vaccination, and (4) promoting judicious antimicrobial drug use.[50] Recognition of antimicrobial resistance patterns may assist physicians in treating patients.[51] DNA chip technology will be used to identify resistance and the most effective and appropriate drug in advance of the initiation of treatment. Worldwide databases will be available to identify emerging epidemics and drug-resistant patterns, and the Web will be used to notify individuals of their need for specific immunizations.

RADIOLOGICAL TECHNOLOGY

In addition to the computerization of the health care encounter, the advances in genomics, and the customization of individual specific drugs and treatment protocol, significant advances in biotechnologies will influence radiological and surgical treatments in the future. Digital x-ray detectors using amorphous silicon technology will result in electronic images, eliminating film processing and storage. This technology will result in electronic archiving, remote digital communication, and computer-aided detection in reviewing clinical images. The image and interpretation could be available in the patient's chart for clinical decision making.

Computer-aided screening and interpretation of x-ray images could have a profound effect on the availability, standardization, and cost of radiological services. There will be significant expansion and advancement in the use of the positron emission tomography (PET) scan. PET scans reveal which area of the brain is responsible for specific functions. This technology could be used not only in the diagnosis of specific disease states but also could be used in patient decision making by identifying a patient's response to a specific treatment option.

A device is currently being developed that integrates PET with computer-assisted x-ray tomography (CT) scans to yield startling images that could improve diagnosis of cancer. CT typically provides very good images of anatomical anomalies, but does not indicate whether disease is present. Conversely, PET shows "hot spots" that physicians can use as markers of disease, but does not indicate from which part of the anatomy the abnormality originates.[52] By combining the two technologies, anatomical and functional images can be viewed as a single image, increasing the accuracy and usefulness of the test.

PDT (photodynamic therapy) is a process in which target cells take up dye and a light source is used to treat the target cells. A new light-emitting diode probe developed under a NASA grant is currently being used for photodynamic brain cancer therapy. The space shuttle Discovery, launched October 29, 1998, had numerous experiments related to treatment of cancer, including: (1) efforts to grow live cells in space using rotating cylinders, or bioreactors, to provide insight into how cancer cells proliferate; (2) experiments to test the effectiveness of microencapsulation of cancer-fighting drugs; and (3) research into the role of the enzyme urokinase in the spread of brain, lung, colon, prostate, and breast cancers.[53] As the international space station is built over the next few years, it will develop into a research laboratory with the potential for increasing our knowledge of the disease process and developing new technologies for use in treatment.

SURGICAL TECHNOLOGY

The field of surgery changed dramatically in 1986 with the introduction of laparoscopic gallbladder surgery. This was the start of minimally invasive and visually enhanced surgery. Virtual reality (VR) can exploit these current trends in miniaturization and set the stage for the coming surgical revolution.

The VR interface is a combination of embedded intelligence, three-dimensional displays, voice-controlled robotic systems, motion-tracking sensors, datagloves, fiberoptic sensors, high-fidelity tactile sensors, and actuators. Combining VR with generic image data and patient-specific data, high-fidelity optical and tactile sensors communicating through high-bandwidth data links will let geographically separated surgeons form virtual teams for telesurgery on distant patients. Virtual humans can be created by taking realistic data from patient-specific CT and MRI images or from databases. The data can be acquired before the operation and combined in surgical simulators for a VR test. MRI-guided surgery allows tracking the path of a surgical instrument using MRI equipment that will allow tissues beyond the surgeon's unaided view to be seen clearly and in detail.

Surgical training simulators will have rule-based judgment, incorporating fuzzy logic in VR-based teaching simulators to allow measurement of a student's or surgeon's performance. Telementoring will use a technique called "deep pixels" that lets every pixel store massive amounts of information, such as anatomic function, color, texture, dynamic movement, physiology parameters, and biochemical values. The organ represented by those pixels could have all the properties of living tissue and permit a person to interact with it as if it were real.[54] Surgical training and ongoing assessment of skills could benefit from these techniques in judging the performances of individuals, and this information could be available over the Internet to aid patients in the selection of their surgeon.

MICROTECHNOLOGY VERSUS NANOTECHNOLOGY

To understand the significance of micro- and nanotechnology, it is helpful to have a sense of the size with which one is dealing. A meter is about 40 inches long. A micro unit (micron) is one millionth of a meter. A nanometer is one billionth of a meter. A human red cell is about 10 micrometers, a bacterium around 1 micrometer. The hemoglobin molecule is 10 nanometers, the glucose molecule about 0.9 nanometer, and a carbon bond about 0.1 nanometer. The double helix of DNA is 2.3 nanometers wide.

Microtechnology is an evolving discipline best illustrated by the expansion of the number of transistors placed on the CPU of Intel chips—increasing from 29,000 on the 8086 chip in 1978 to over 3 million on the Pentium II chip. By the year 2000, the newest computer chips are expected to contain from 50 to 100 million transistors per chip and be capable of executing more than 2 billion instructions per second.

Techniques developed for producing computer chips are now being applied to the development of microscale devices, sensors, and chemical analyzers. As a result, small motors, optical and electrochemical detectors, gears, bearings, pipets, pumps, relays, solenoids, and valves have been produced.[55] Personal wearable health monitors of minute size will be connected to computers by infrared data transfer to continuously monitor critical functions. With built-in protocols, the monitors can be manipulated to adjust treatment as needed.

Nanotechnology is the precise manipulation of individual atoms and molecules to create larger structures. Since the late 1970s, K. Eric Drexler has argued that the absolute control of matter at the smallest scale is an achievable goal and would lead to molecular manufacturing with the aid of multitudes of submicroscopic "assemblers." The goal of nanotechnology is the custom design and production of molecules. The construction of general-purpose assemblers will enable us to build molecular structures. They can also produce assemblers identical to themselves called "replicators." With the production of replicators, mass production of the desired molecular structure is possible.

The development of the scanning tunneling microscope in 1981 gave the first images of individual atoms. Coupled with the development of the atomic force microscope, this has brought scientists closer to the capability to study and manipulate molecular structures. Some of the building blocks have already been identified. A new form of carbon molecule shaped like a soccer ball, called a *buckyball*, is one of those building blocks. Elongated tubes of carbon called *buckytubes* would be used to form nanotubes that could be used to transfer molecular structures in and out of cells. Biomolecules with light-addressed memory modules could be used to build biocomputers.

Among the fruits of nanotechnology may be tiny electronic devices such as ultrasmall sensors no thicker than a large protein molecule. A family of scanning-probe microscopes attached to a computer would create *in vivo* nanoscopes for the investigation of biological processes inside the cells of living animals. Microscopic robotic devices will patrol the human body, identify abnormal molecular structure such as cancer cells, and repair or destroy them. Nanoassemblers could be designed to produce a wide variety of replacement tissues, replacing rather than transplanting whole organs. "Within fifty to a hundred years, a new class of organisms is likely to emerge . . . and 'evolve' into something other than their original form."[56]

THE ANTITECHNOLOGY REVOLUTION

As great advancements are made in the identification and utilization of emerging technologies, an increasing segment of the population is looking for a more basic approach to managing its own health. A recent survey shows a significant increase in the use of alternative medicine, with at least one out of 16 people using alternative therapies during the previous year, increasing from 33.8 percent in 1990 to 42.1 percent in 1997.[57] The most rapidly increasing therapies include herbal medicine, massage therapy, megavitamins, self-help groups, folk remedies, energy healing, and homeopathy. Estimated expenditures for alternative medicine professional services increased 45.2 percent between 1990 and 1997 and were estimated at $21.2 billion in 1997, with at least $12.2 billion paid out-of-pocket. Research in alternative medicine will help identify what is safe and effective and will further the understanding of biology. "Alternative medicine is here to stay. It is no longer an option to ignore it or treat it as something outside the normal processes of science and medicine. The challenge is to move forward carefully, using both reason and wisdom, as we attempt to separate the pearls from the mud."[58]

CONCLUSION

The challenge facing medicine is to incorporate the advances in technology into a user-friendly interface that allows individuals to participate as equal partners in their health care decision making. A free flow of information will allow informed decision making on the part of the providers and the recipients of health care. "Mass customization" will result from mining worldwide databases searching for best practices, and this will be combined with patient-specific genetic data and disease-specific data to formulate the best treatment options based on patient preference.

References

1. David M. Eddy, *Clinical Decision-Making: From Theory to Practice* (Sudbury, MA: Jones and Bartlett Publishers, 1996), p. 8.

2. David Eddy, *A Manual for Assessing Health Practices & Designing Practice Policies: The Explicit Approach* (Philadelphia: American College of Physicians, 1992), p. 18.

3. Gilad J. Kuperman, Reed M. Gardner, and T. Allan Pryor, *HELP: A Dynamic Hospital Information System* (New York: Springer-Verlag, 1991).

4. Michael W. Davis, *Computerizing Healthcare Information* (New York: McGraw-Hill, 1998), p. 5.

5. Sam H. Schmitt, "Technological Front-Runners or Sheep to the Slaughter?" *Managed Healthcare* (August 1998): 36–38.

6. Jennifer Day, "Tracking the Trends in Healthcare Information Systems," *Healthcare Business Monthly* (August 1998): 12–13.

7. Howard Kim, "Patients May Carry Records on Their Wrist," *American Medical News* (June 15/22, 1998): 43.

8. Patrice Degoulet and Marius Fieschi, *Introduction to Clinical Informatics* (New York: Springer, 1997) p. 195.

9. Kathryn Trombature, "Opinion: A Question of Privacy'" *American Medical News* 41, no. 32 (August 24, 1998): 21.

10. American Medical Association (AMA) Board of Trustees: "Report on Patient Privacy and Confidentiality," presented by Thomas R. Reardon, AMA House of Delegates meeting, Chicago (June 12-14, 1998).

11. Diane S. Schneidman, *The Medical Records Confidentiality Issue: An Overview* (Chicago: Bulletin of the American College of Surgeons, August 1998), p. 20.

12. Theresa Falzone, "Centralized Patient Information Database . . . or Databuse?" *Healthcare Business Monthly* (July 1998): 14–21.

13. Geri Aston, "Privacy of Records in Doubt," *American Medical News* 41, no.30 (August 10, 1998): 1, 48.

14. Deloitte & Touche Consulting Group, "Industry Watch," *Health Management Technology* (August 1998)

15. Larry Stevens and Kitty Meek, "High-Tech House Calls," *American Medical News* (September 14, 1998): 30–34.

16. Gary Baldwin, "Web Doc," *American Medical News* (July 27, 1998): 26–27.

17. Briggs T. Pille, "The Use of the Internet in Healthcare," *Michigan Healthcare* 3, no. 8 (August 1998): 1, 18.

18. Charles Cohen, "The New Black Bag," *Net Discovery* (summer 1998): 1013.

19. Don Tapscott, *Growing Up Digital, The Rise of the Net Generation* (New York, McGraw-Hill, 1998).

20. Surveys, "Physicians Say Internet Information Improves Care," *Health Management Technology* (August 1998): 8.

21. Sandra Guy, "Conference Highlights: Growing Reach of the Internet," *American Medical News* 41, No. 43 (November 16, 1998): 29.

22. Abigail Green, "Doctor.com," *Net Discovery* (summer 1998): 6–9.

23. Gerald Miller, "Supplying Provider Data via the Internet," *Health Management Technology* (August 1998): 42–44.

24. Gary Baldwin, "System Makes It Easier to Link Patients to Clinical Trials," *American Medical News* 41, no. 43 (November 16, 1998): 27–28.

25. Gary Baldwin, "Web Rx," *American Medical News* 41, no. 29 (August 3, 1998): 29–31.

26. Howard Kim, "CME: A Whole New World (Wide Web)," *American Medical News* 41, no. 32 (August 24, 1998): 23–24.

27. Gary Baldwin, "Intranet Links Emergency Departments," *American Medical News* 41, no. 31 (August 17, 1998): 30.

28. Tim Harris, "Correspondence: in Defense of Genomics," *Nature Biotechnology* 15 (September 1997): 820.

29. A. S. Roses et al., "Measuring the Genetic Contribution of APOE in Late-Onset Alzheimer Disease (AD)," *American Journal of Human Genetics* 57 (1995): (suppl) A202.

30. Ekaterina Rogaeva et al., "Evidence for an Alzheimer Disease Susceptibility Locus on Chromosome 12 and for Further Locus Heterogeneity," *Journal of the American Medical Association* 280, no 7 (August 19, 1998): 614–17.

31. Charles F. Sing et al., "Biological Complexity and Strategies for Finding DNA Variations Responsible for Inter-Individual Variation in Risk of a Common Chronic Disease, Coronary Artery Disease," *Annals of Medicine* 24 (1992): 539–47.

32. C. F. Sing et al., "Application of Cladistics to the Analysis of Genotype-Phenotype Relationships," *European Journal of Epidemiology* 8 no. 2 (suppl. 1992): 3–9.

33. Robert F. Service, "DNA Chips Survey an Entire Genome," *Science* 281 (August 21, 1998): 1122.

34. Bill Benett et al., "A Miniature Analytical Instrument for Nucleic Acids Based on Micromachined Silicon Reaction Chambers," *Analytical Chemistry* 70, no. 5 (March 1, 1998): 918–22.

35. Jeremy Rifkin, *The Biotech Century* (New York: Penguin Putman Inc., 1998) pp. 8–9.

36. George Poste, "Moleculare Medicine and Information-Based Targeted Healthcare," *Nature Biotechnology* 16 (supplement 1998): 19–21.

37. Thomas Chang, MD, PhD, director of the Artifical Cells and Organs Research Center at McGill University, *AMN* (November 16, 1998): 31.

38. Aris Persidis, "Biotechnologies to Watch," *Nature Biotechnology* 15 (December 1997): 1409–11.

39. Jonathan H. Lin, "Divining and Altering the Future: Implications from the Human Genome Project," *Journal of the American Medical Association* 280 (1998): 1532.

40. H. Gilbert Welch and Wylie Burke, "Uncertainties in Genetic Testing for Chronic Disease," *Journal of the American Medical Association* 280 (1998): 1525–27.

41. Sarah Klein, "Stricter Patient Privacy Controls Urged," *American Medical News* (July 6, 1998): 14.

42. Tim Friend, "Drug Revolution Shakes Industry," *USA TODAY* (November 24, 1998): 17A.

43. Tim Friend, "Technologies Help Scientists Develop Drugs More Quickly," *USA TODAY* (November 24, 1998): 18A.

44. Council on Scientific Affairs, "Epidemic Infectious Disease Risks: Striving for Perspective," *Journal of the American Medical Association* 275, no. 3 (1996): 181.

45. Robert W. Pinner et al., "Trends in Infectious Diseases Mortality in the United States," *Journal of the American Medical Association* 275, no. 3 (January 17, 1996): 189.

46. Laurie Garrett, *The Coming Plague; Newly Emerging Diseases in a World out of Balance* (New York: Penguin Books, 1995).

47. Michael J. Kozal et el., "Extensive Polymorphisms Observed in HIV-1 Clade B Protease Gene Using High-Density Oligonucleotide Arrays," *Nature Medicine* 2, no. 7 (July 1996): 753–59.

48. Dale J. Hu et al., "The Emerging Genetic Diversity of HIV," *Journal of the American Medical Association* 275, no. 3 (January 17, 1996): 210–15.

49. Donald A. Goldmann et al., "Strategies to Prevent and Control the Emergence and Spread of Antimicrobial-Resistant Microorganisms in Hospitals," *Journal of the American Medical Association* 275 (1996): 234–40.

50. Daniel B. Jernigan et al., "Minimizing the Impact of Drug-Resistant Stretococcus Pneumoniae (DRSP)," *Journal of the American Medical Association* 275, no. 3 (January 17, 1996): 206.

51. Joseph F. Plouffe et al., "Bacteremia with Streptococcus Pneumoniae: Implications for Therapy and Prevention," *Journal of the American Medical Association* 275, no. 3 (January 17, 1996): 194.

52. Mark Moran, "Are Two Scanners Better Than One?" *American Medical News* (September 21, 1998): 39–40.

53. Mark Moran, "Scientists Bring Space Technologies Down to Earth," *American Medical News* 41, no. 43 (November 16, 1998): 30, 36.

54. Richard M. Satava and Shaun B. Jones, "Medicine Beyond the Year 2000," *Caduceus* 13, no. 2 (autumn 1997): 49–64.

55. C. A. Burtis, "Technological Trends in Clinical Laboratory Science," *Clinical Biochemistry* 28 (June 1995): 213–19.

56. B. C. Crandall, *NANOtechnology, Molecular Speculations on Global Abundance* (Cambridge, MA: The MIT Press, 1998), p. 28.

57. David M. Eisenberg et al., "Trends in Alternative Medicine Use in the United States 1990–1997," *Journal of the American Medical Association* 280 (1998): 1569–75.

58. Wayne B. Jonas, "Alternative Medicine—Learning From the Past, Examining the Present, Advancing to the Future," *Journal of the American Medical Association* 280 (1998): 1617.

CHAPTER 9

IMPACT OF TECHNOLOGY ON NURSING CARE

Margaret L. Campbell, RN

T o me, the future described by David Ellis in part 1 of this book is plausible and will have a significant impact on the manner in which care is provided to patients by nurses, particularly in the high-technology world of the critical care unit (CCU). In this chapter I describe current practice and contrast it with my imaginings of the potential care milieu in 2030 employing projected technologies and assists. My aim is not only to capture the promise but also the possible liabilities of these wonders.

Critical care units have been in existence since the 1960s and are designed to provide intensive monitoring (physical and automated), life-sustaining therapies, and a small nurse-to-patient ratio for patients experiencing or at risk for life-threatening illnesses or injuries. These units illustrate the health care technology explosion.

Advances in critical care technologies over the past 30 years (smaller, integrated, and rapid) have allowed therapies that were once only the purview of the CCU to be taken into long-term care facilities and patient homes. For example, patients who are dependent on mechanical ventilators now have the opportunity to move about freely, even to travel, since the ventilator and its battery pack are small, portable, and user-friendly.

It is likely that some of the forecasted changes for hospital care proposed by Ellis will first be found in critical care units. I will provide a characterization of current practice in CCU contrasted with projections for 2030. For both the current illustration and the future characterization, imagine a critical care unit with a patient census of 12 critically ill patients in various stages of acuity requiring various intensities of life support.

STAFFING/RESPONSIBILITIES

It is 1999 at Somewhere Memorial Hospital. The care team for the next eight hours consists of six registered nurses, one respiratory therapist, one clinical pharmacist, two nurse's aides, and one housekeeper/food service technician.

Each registered nurse has overall responsibility for the care of two patients and delegates tasks to the nurse's aides and housekeepers. The major RN responsibilities include: physical exam; monitoring and analysis of hemodynamic, pulmonary, and metabolic data; initiation and maintenance of nursing and prescribed medical therapies; drug administration and titration; patient teaching and counseling; and family support. The RN collaborates with the patient's primary physician to plan and deliver the requisite care.

The nurse's aides, under the supervision of the RN, provide basic patient care such as bathing, linen changes, simple dressing changes, specimen collection, specimen delivery, and pharmacy or blood bank materials retrieval. A complete bath and linen change requires approximately 20 minutes and one aide if the patient can participate in the bath by turning independently. The task requires two or more nurses or aides if the patient is completely dependent.

The respiratory therapist provides aerosolized breathing treatments, analyzes arterial blood gas samples in the minilab adjacent to the CCU, and monitors and adjusts mechanical ventilators according to the medical plan. Regular tubing changes and preventive maintenance of the ventilator are performed each day.

The clinical pharmacist makes rounds with the intensivist and staff nurses and provides drug information and consultation, analyzes laboratory pharmacokinetics, and facilitates rapid drug delivery from the pharmacy adjacent to the CCU. The pharmacist responds to pages throughout the day as drug information is required and is a member of the emergency response team when cardiopulmonary resuscitation is being performed anywhere in the hospital.

The housekeeper/food service technician provides basic support such as laundry delivery, unit cleaning, food tray delivery and pickup, and other basic tasks assigned by the RNs. This unskilled aide may also be used to facilitate heavy tasks such as lifting or turning dependent patients, retrieving supplies from other parts of the hospital, and delivering specimens.

Other disciplines and technicians, such as chaplains, physical therapists, or radiology technicians, intervene with the patients throughout the day as needed. The RN attempts to coordinate all these activities and interventions to ensure patient stability and energy conservation.

Today, as illustrated, care in the CCU is labor intensive, costly, and requires collaboration among a large number of disciplines and individuals. It has been characterized as fragmented. A recent cost-saving strategy is aimed at reducing the number of high-salaried RNs and replacing them with unlicensed, low-salaried nurse's aides. The strategy has raised fears about inadequate patient outcomes because the hospitalized patient's needs are complex and aides are only trained in rudimentary tasks.

Improvements such as those forecast may contribute to decreased labor intensity and more comprehensive, inexpensive care. It is also likely that the number of RNs needed to deliver care will be fewer as computers and robots complement human skills.

Forecast

The year is 2030, the place is Somewhere-Someplace-Anotherplace Memorial General Community Hospital and Health System (SSAMGCHHS). In the critical care unit it is 0700. For the next eight hours, the care team consists of two registered nurses, a biomedical engineer, and six robots.

Each RN has overall responsibility for six patients and attends to monitoring and analyzing patient data generated continuously by the robots and computers. The plan of care is adjusted in collaboration with the intensivist, who makes rounds with the RNs from his office in which he has access to all the patient data. The RN determines which patient tasks will be completed by herself and which by the robot, and she engages in patient counseling and teaching and family support.

The robots obtain, analyze, and synthesize hemodynamic, pulmonary, and metabolic patient data; provide basic and skilled care; and clean the unit. They also perform respiratory therapies and pharmaceutical analysis and drug delivery. The biomedical engineer provides preventive maintenance to the robots and troubleshoots problems.

Fewer human staff will reduce the cost of care delivery and decrease the amount of service fragmentation. The robots are likely to be able to perform multiple tasks simultaneously and generate highly reliable and objective clinical data. Caution will need to be exercised in designing care delivery models so that they do not rely too heavily on robots with an insufficient number of supportive human personnel.

Many aspects of caring for sick humans relies on subjective responses to subtle signs and cues that may be beyond the capacity of automated devices to recognize and analyze.

REPORTING/COMMUNICATING

In 1999, the new shift begins with each offgoing staff nurse giving a verbal report, one at a time, to the oncoming team about the patients she or he was responsible for on the previous shift. Information includes the patient's name, age, bed number, medical diagnoses, medical treatments, nursing problems, nursing treatments, and information about the family. The facts are illustrated by anecdotes, and occasional humorous characterizations are shared. The oncoming team takes note of pertinent information with paper and pen. Each report requires three to five minutes of information sharing, both relevant and superfluous, and the entire reporting about all 12 patients takes about an hour.

Forecast

In 2030, the offgoing nurse downloads patient data from the six robots to a central viewing area. These data have been automatically synthesized to exclude clinically redundant or irrelevant facts. The computer has also generated a care plan for the next eight hours based on these data, with assignments for each of the robots, and prioritized a list of responsibilities for the RNs.

The oncoming team projects the downloaded data onto a central screen for simultaneous viewing and scrolls through the data and projected care plans and responsibilities. The computer recognizes and responds to verbal requests for more data or more detail when the nurses seek more information. The synthesized report is prepared in less than 5 minutes for 12 complex patients. Review, integration, and modification by the oncoming RNs requires about 20 minutes for 12 patients.

A significant amount of time can be saved with better integration of computer systems in routine unit operations. Verbal reports take more time than scrolling through a synthesized printed report. In addition, the data synthesized by the computer will be more objective and the potential for errors due to oversight or transcription mistakes will be eliminated.

PATIENT CARE

In 1999, a complete physical exam by the RN at the beginning of a shift takes approximately 20 minutes for each patient and includes evaluation and adjustment of all monitoring devices, invasive catheters, and infusions. Less complete reevaluations are performed hourly and when there are changes in a patient's condition. The electrocardiogram and hemodynamic monitors are recalibrated at the beginning of each shift and whenever irregular or inconsistent data are displayed. A paper recording of the waveforms is collected each shift and pasted into the patient's chart. Data obtained from the patient's examination and the monitors are recorded by hand on a paper flowsheet. Each flowsheet represents one 24-hour interval and becomes a part of the permanent paper record. Narrative notes document other aspects of care relevant to the patient's nursing problem list.

Medical prescriptions for medications, diagnostic tests, and respiratory treatments are reviewed and forwarded to the relevant departments via internal fax machines. Medications delivered by pharmacy technicians are verified for accuracy and administered. Patients are observed for drug effects, which are documented in the medical record.

Some diagnostic exams are conducted at the bedside using portable equipment, such as radiographs, electrocardiograms, electroencephalograms, and endoscopic examinations. More complex tests, such as angiograms, CAT scans, and MRI scans, require moving the patient from the CCU via bed or stretcher to the location of the test. The patient is escorted to the test by at least one RN, one respiratory therapist, and a transportation technician. The other RNs provide coverage to the traveling RN's other patient during her absence from the CCU. In some hospitals, a special team of RNs is responsible for providing patient escorts for tests, allowing the CCU RNs to remain behind to care for the other unit patients.[1]

Throughout all the care delivery, patients are spoken to, explanations of care are offered, questions are answered, and teaching is provided if relevant. Patients' families are supported during their visits and given information about the patients' progress and prognosis. In some cases, preprinted educational or other supportive materials are provided to the patient or the family.

Forecast

In 2030, most of the routine patient care is delivered by robots, with the RNs monitoring progress and interrupting programming when the patient care must be done by the RN. The robots continuously feed patient data to a central record, which can be accessed from anywhere in the care network, including the physician office, pharmacy, laboratory, kitchen, finance department, and so on. The RNs monitor the data for clinical clarity and relevance and edit by dictating to speech-recognizing computers.

Many clinical tasks are capably performed by the robots, including placement of venous or arterial access devices, sampling body fluids, recording vital signs, auscultating lung sounds, manipulating intravenous fluids, administering routine and emergency medications, administering blood products, bathing, weighing, and changing linen. The RNs monitor the care provided by the robots and are prepared to replace them in situations calling for human sensitivity.

In spite of the ability to recognize human voices and translate from many languages, the voice recognition technology remains incapable of interpreting nonverbal communication, with the exception of international sign language. Critically ill patients with artificial airways can only communicate nonverbally through a number of methods using language boards and hand signals. It is common for nurses to need to read lips when the critically ill patient is too sick to make use of language devices. Lip-reading comprehension is complicated by the presence of oral airway devices and demands a certain finesse from the staff to be able to interpret the patient's communication. Finally, the communication itself may be delusional, confused, or incomprehensible as a result of impaired consciousness. The subtlety of this form of interpreting patient communication lies beyond the skill of robots and computers.

Data from the robots are collected continuously and have a higher degree of validity and reliability than data collected manually, as was the case in 1999. Artifacts and irregularities are deleted from the analysis and there is more consistency. In addition, drug administration and infusion devices are an integral component of the robot, allowing for rapid adjustments of medications to correspond to continuous data interpretation.

CARDIOPULMONARY RESUSCITATION

In 1999, cardiac monitors can recognize dysrrhythmia patterns with some degree of accuracy. An alarm cues the RN that there may be a life-threatening cardiac rhythm, which the RN validates by viewing the monitor screen and quickly assessing the patient for loose monitoring leads or other causes of artifact and false alarms. Emergency drugs are administered according to protocol if the dysrrhythmia is valid. The Code Blue emergency response team is alerted if the emergency persists and cardiac arrest occurs or is imminent. Physicians, residents-in-training, medical students, respiratory therapists, a pharmacist, and a nursing supervisor will all respond to the call for emergency support. A crash cart containing resuscitation devices, drugs, and a defibrillator/cardioverter is wheeled to the bedside. A chaotic appearance is in fact illustrative of a number of disciplines engaged in multiple rescue-oriented tasks simultaneously.

Forecast

In 2030, the automated robot system detects the patient's cardiac performance and rhythm continuously. Changes signifying a life-threatening dysrrhythmia prompt an automatic administration of the appropriate rescue drug from a reservoir in the robot. Cardioversion or defibrillation can also be generated immediately when indicated without having to wheel a crash cart to the bedside. This more immediate response to life-threatening changes improves postresuscitation morbidity and mortality.

TEACHING/COUNSELING

In 1999 the RN provides teaching, counseling, and family support functions. Patient teaching is supported by generic educational pamphlets and materials generated for the person with an average reading comprehension. Some materials are available in Spanish, but most are only available in English. RNs will attempt to tailor the information provided to patients or their families by giving consideration to educational level, reading comprehension, and the deleterious effects of illness and stress. Critically ill patients and their stressed families require frequent reinforcement of information because illness and stress interfere with information processing.

Forecast

In 2030, teaching, counseling, and family support functions are done by the RN with support from the computer. The computer automatically transcribes the person-to-person discussion into the language most comprehensible to the patient or family at an age-relevant and culturally relevant level and provides the family with an individualized takeaway document.

KNOWLEDGE ATTAINMENT

In 1999, one of the patients in the CCU has a rare diagnosis for which the staff has no previous experience. The critical care nurse educator and clinical nurse specialist are called to provide resource materials about this patient's unique care needs. A review of current critical care nursing textbooks discloses no information about this diagnosis. A Medline library search identifies two case reports in journals, but they are not immediately available. The librarian will seek an interlibrary loan and the articles should be available to the CCU staff within a week. A query for information is posted to two critical care discussion group listservs, but a reply will not be forthcoming until a group member with information reads and replies to the post. A search for information on the Internet reveals one case report from Berlin, but the abstract is not translated into English. The staff are left with designing care for this patient according to clinical judgment and intuition.

Forecast

In 2030, one of the patients has a rare and complex diagnosis. Few nurses have ever had an opportunity to see this phenomenon or provide care for patients experiencing it. The RNs at SSAMGCHHS are able to chat online with nurses internationally with automatic language translation and gather information about the experiences of 15 other RNs who had encountered this rare diagnosis. This evolving chat resulted in the RNs having the collective wisdom and experience of caring for 15 similar patients instead of just one. The chat discussion is picked up by an online clinical journal and transcribed into an analysis and discussion of case reports for archive and reaccess purposes by others at some future time.

PALLIATION AND PRESENCE

In 1999, one of the patients has multiple-system organ failure and is not expected to survive. Continued, aggressive therapy is not predicted to change the outcome. Clinical judgment, physician experience, and evidence-based reports in the literature guide the determination of the poor prognosis. In some facilities, computer programs or illness severity scales are used to validate the predictions of the clinical staff.[2,3]

The decision is made by the CCU physician and staff nurse with the patient's family to change the goal of treatment to comfort measures only. Thus, the emphasis of the patient's remaining hours of care will be on palliation and support of his family. Critical care interventions no longer relevant are discontinued, particularly if they merely prolong dying or are potential sources of discomfort. The patient is observed for signs of distress, which is palliated with medication and other strategies. The family sits at the bedside and is supported in its grief by the RNs and the hospital chaplain.

Subtle, subjective responses are interpreted by the RN to represent presumed distress. The patient is no longer able to provide a self-report about how he is feeling. The RN validates her impression with the patient's wife, who is at the bedside with their children. The family also believes that the patient is uncomfortable, and the RN provides a bolus of an analgesic.

Forecast

In 2030, the computer provides morbidity and mortality estimations on a daily basis or when queried by synthesizing the patient's responses and correlating them with evidence-based outcomes. The clinical staff are prompted to begin discussions with the patient or surrogates about end-of-life decisions when the probability of patient death is greater than 50 percent.

When the decision is made to focus on comfort, the computer/ robot automatically reduces superfluous or uncomfortable interventions.

The RN retains responsibility for assessing and responding to patient distress, because this requires a more subjective appraisal of the patient's responses.

Counseling and providing emotional support to the family are also in the purview of the RN because robots/computers are unable to demonstrate empathy (remember HAL).

REHABILITATION

In 1999, considerations for patient rehabilitation are integrated into the plan of care. The RN collaborates with the physical therapist to determine the patient's ability to participate in physical therapy. They rely on clinical judgment and the patient's examination before and during the therapy. During a critical illness, maintaining a balance between the positive effects of rehabilitative strategies and the need to avoid fatigue and promote energy conservation requires careful consideration.

In most hospitals, the physical therapy department operates during the day on weekdays only. Thus, patients receive physical therapy during the busiest and most fatiguing time of the day. Therapies are not provided if the patient is receiving some other treatment or is too sick or tired to benefit.

Forecast

In 2030, the automated robot/computer delivery system incorporates rehabilitative strategies into the daily care. The computer measures muscle tone, performance, patient fatigue, and energy balance and adjusts the therapy accordingly. Therapy is provided by the computer at any time of the day or night according to the patient's abilities and needs.

DISCHARGE/AMBULATORY FOLLOW-UP

In 1999, a patient has improved to the point that critical monitoring is not needed. A transfer from the CCU to a general care unit occurs. When the patient no longer requires hospital-level care, a discharge is coordinated. Patients may go home, to a skilled nursing facility, or to an inpatient rehabilitation facility. A handwritten hospital course summary is forwarded to the skilled nursing or rehabilitation facility. A discharge summary is dictated by the discharging physician and a copy is sent to the patient's primary physician.

Patients who go home receive discharge instructions from the RN. They include directions about activity, diet, medications, and follow-up appointments with physicians or therapists in the ambulatory setting. A handwritten discharge instruction sheet is taken by the patient to reinforce the verbal instructions. Patients with complex ongoing care needs in the home will be seen by home care nurses, therapists, and technicians. Referrals to home care agencies are made prior to discharge and durable medical equipment is ordered and delivered to the home prior to the patient's leaving the hospital. Hospitals employ discharge planners, also known as case managers, to facilitate a timely move from the hospital to the home or long-term care facility with all relevant referrals and supports in place.

Some patients lack a primary care provider and at the next accident or illness may not be seen at the same facility. Hospitals will share summaries of previous hospitalizations after the patient gives consent for the medical record to be copied and delivered. Clearly, delays in obtaining medical histories can compromise care, morbidity, and mortality.

Forecast

In 2030, the computer regularly adjusts the intensity of acute patient care according to patient responses. Readiness for hospital discharge is predicted along with relevant referrals and orders for durable medical equipment. The discharge summary is integrated into the patient's smart card, allowing access to future care providers without delays.

NURSING EDUCATION AND TRAINING

In 1999, a state license to practice as an RN is awarded after two, three, or four years of study in an associate, diploma, or baccalaureate program.[4] A national examination (called *boards*) sets the standard for licensure. The knowledge base for nursing practice is derived from nursing science; philosophy and ethics; and physical, economic, biomedical, behavioral, and social sciences.

Advanced practice nurses have acquired the knowledge base and practice experience to prepare for specialization, expansion, and advancement in practice generally after completion of a master's degree. Advanced practice nursing has evolved in the roles of nurse practitioner, clinical nurse specialist, nurse midwife, and nurse anesthetist.

Forecast

In 2030, an RN will be prepared at the master's level for entry into practice. In addition to the coursework previously described, nursing students will need to be prepared in computer technologies and in working with robots.

SUMMARY

The 2030 scenario I have painted is less aggressive than David Ellis would probably envision. It still includes hospitals and humans as a vital part of the health care encounter, though there are fewer humans who are trained at a higher level to focus on higher-level nursing tasks, tasks involving human intuition and the human touch, which no machine can emulate.

References and Note

1. H. E. Stearley, "Patient Outcomes: Intrahospital Transportation and Monitoring of Critically Ill Patients by a Specially Trained ICU Nursing Staff," *American Journal of Critical Care* 7 (1998): 282–87.

2. W. A. Knaus et al., "APACHE II: A Severity of Disease Classification System," *Critical Care Medicine* 13 (1985): 818–29.

3. J. E. Zimmerman et al., "Evaluation of Acute Physiology and Chronic Health Evaluation III Predictions of Hospital Mortality in an Independent Database," *Critical Care Medicine* 26 (1998): 1317–26.

4. South Dakota is the only state that requires a baccalaureate degree for RN licensure. Since 1965, the American Nurses' Association has consistently affirmed the baccalaureate degree in nursing as the preferred requirement for basic nursing practice.

CHAPTER 10

HOSPITALS AND THE FORCES OF CHANGE

Brian E. Peters, MHSA

T he 1990s have not been kind to the core business of the nation's community hospitals. Virtually every yardstick of inpatient activity has shown dramatic decline throughout the decade: acute care admissions, hospital days, average length of stay, and even the number of staffed inpatient beds have all been reduced in the face of upheavals in the industry. Perhaps the most telling statement: in a U.S. national Inter-Study survey asking health maintenance organization (HMO) executives to identify their top reasons for achieving financial success over the past year, "favorable hospital utilization" was the top response.[1]

THE CHANGES AFFECTING HOSPITALS

The forces acting on the American hospital are many and complex, but they are worth examining if one is to fully understand the impact that the emerging technology age will have on this central component of our health care delivery system. These forces include, but certainly are not limited to a dramatic aging of the population, an increase in the use of managed care by public payers (Medicare and Medicaid), a private sector that is becoming more aggressive and sophisticated in its negotiations with providers over quality and price, and the rise of consumerism as the general public takes a much more active role in its own care. These specific changes are taking place against an overarching shift away from a medical model to a healthy communities model in American health care.

In 1996, 12.8 percent of the U.S. population was age 65 or older; 5.7 percent was 75 or older; and 1.4 percent was 85 or older. By the year 2030, fully 20 percent of the population will be age 65 or older; 9.2 percent will be 75 or older, and 2.4 percent will be 85 or older.[2] The financial implications of this trend are troubling, even in the shorter term: total mandatory Medicare spending is projected to more than double, from $196.1 billion in 1996 to $463 billion in 2006.[3]

For years, federal and state governments essentially sat on the sidelines and watched the private sector achieve remarkable success in containing health benefit costs through managed care; in both 1995 and 1996, the average HMO premium in the United States actually declined.[4] Medicare's interest in expanding managed care enrollment among its beneficiaries comes at a unique time in American history, as the baby boomers are set to retire and place an unprecedented strain on the social welfare system. Compared to their predecessors, this new cohort of Medicare eligibles has a greater familiarity—and presumably more comfort—with HMOs. Their former employers, seeking to take advantage of the accounting magic of FASB 106, are also likely to encourage these new retirees to join Medicare HMOs.

In the absence of a strong lobbying group representing the affected party, the rise of Medicaid managed care has been meteoric in comparison with Medicare. With the subtlety of a freight train, many states have implemented managed care programs for the poor that radically change the patient-provider relationship as well as the prevailing reimbursement model.

Large, multistate employers are increasingly questioning the variability in medical practice. Ford, Chrysler, and General Motors want to know why the c-section rate for its employees is significantly higher in one state than it is in another and why average length of stay for its employees is higher than the length of stay for other patients in the same hospital. Such variability does not exist among any of its other suppliers.

These large employers, armed with the best available clinical outcomes and financial data, are becoming integrally involved in improving the performance of hospitals, physicians, and health plans. But they are not alone. The emergence of employer coalitions has also given small and medium-sized companies the market clout to aggressively engage in provider profiling and direct contracting.

Finally, the passive patient is rapidly becoming an endangered species and could be extinct by the end of the next decade. At the macro level, the great debate over health care reform that was perhaps the defining characteristic of Bill Clinton's first term in office served to shine the intense spotlight of national media attention on the delivery and financing system. This prolonged debate educated Americans on both the positive and negative aspects of our system and the fragility of coverage even in the midst of a strong economy.

Much more important, the explosion of user-friendly information technology—most notably the Internet—has allowed consumers to readily access information about their particular ailment, the available treatment regimens, cutting-edge surgical techniques and pharmaceuticals, and in some cases the relative performance of different providers. The end result, appropriately termed "popping the God bubble" by the Institute for the Future, is that the treatment decisions of physicians are no longer going unquestioned, and patients are taking a much more active role in their own care.

LEAVING BEHIND THE MEDICAL MODEL?

On a higher plane, all of these changes are secondary in their scope and impact to another fundamental shift that is occurring today. The medical model, whereby health is defined merely as the absence of disease, was predicated on sick individuals showing up at the provider's doorstep and receiving treatment. This model has dominated the delivery of health care in the United States throughout the twentieth century, and hospitals were—and continue in most markets to be—at the epicenter. In 1997, approximately $416 billion—fully 35.5 percent of U.S. health expenditures—was claimed by hospitals. The next largest share went to physicians, who received approximately 19.1 percent of health expenditures.[5]

The "medical arms race" was a natural part of this model, as competing hospitals battled to have the latest hi-tech equipment available in their facilities. The extent of this competition was made evident as health policy analysts compared the American and Canadian systems during the short-lived public outcry for government-run universal health care in the early 1990s. The dramatic difference between the United States and our northern neighbor (and the rest of the industrialized world, for that matter) became strikingly clear; there were (and are today) more MRI machines in Detroit than in all of Canada.[6]

This type of technology-based competition, prevalent in many other industries, was restricted by a formal mechanism unique to the health care field: the development of state-level certificate of need (CON) laws. These laws, supported by large employers who viewed them as one of the only tangible tools to contain health care costs, focused on what was perceived as excessive duplication of big-ticket equipment and services like computerized tomography scanners, magnetic resonance imaging machines, positron emission tomography scanners, lithotripters, megavoltage radiation therapy, organ transplantation, air ambulances, cardiac catheterization, and open heart surgery.

If the comparative studies of national health care systems clarified anything, it was the fact that Americans want ready access to state-of-the-art technology and services. More than anything else, what killed popular enthusiasm for a Canadian- or British-style health care system in the United States was the realization that long waiting lists (queues in the U.K.) for certain services are a fact of life in those systems, and some services simply are not available at all.

But despite an endless progression of advancements in medical technology, many would argue that the quality of life for most Americans has not improved at the same rate. It is possible that in many respects, technology development outpaces the wisdom to deal with it. The most modern medical services are not enough; we need to promote health as well as use science and technology. As managed care continues to take root, providers will increasingly have a financial incentive to blend the medical model with the healthy communities model—to be proactive in partnering with schools, churches, and other community resources to dramatically improve health status and thereby minimize hospitalizations.

Ian Morrison, president of the Institute for the Future, has often challenged the hospital industry not to become the railways of the 1990s, a reference to the critical mistake of the American railway industry at the end of the last century in failing to define their business appropriately. While the railways should have defined themselves more broadly as being in the *transportation* business, the modern hospital industry should define itself as being in the *health* business—not just inpatient care.

Indeed, this emerging model calls for a certain degree of decentralization of the delivery system. In truth, it has been suggested that the medical delivery system (doctors, hospitals, and the like) contributes no more than 10 percent to the intricate puzzle that comprises health status.[7] The other components include environmental conditions (like a clean water supply), genetics, and personal lifestyle behaviors.

It is the latter component that has provided eternal frustration for health care providers, and it is a frustration that is not likely to be reduced by the introduction of new technologies. As long as smoking, alcohol and substance abuse, obesity, violence, sexually transmitted disease, and other lifestyle-related factors continue to exist, health care providers will be fighting an uphill battle. As Leland Kaiser once remarked, "Health is an outcome condition which occurs when everything else [outside the medical delivery system] in the community is working well."

In a rapidly aging society, the benefits of the healthy communities movement will be significant in the years to come. Within the Medicare program, a tiny fraction of the beneficiaries—approximately 3 percent—account for some 39 percent of total Medicare spending.[8] If the new cohort of Medicare eligibles enters the system with a high incidence of chronic disease resulting from adverse lifestyle choices, the system will be further pressured to balance its funding stream with provider payments.

For any provider or health plan that is assuming financial risk under a capitated contract, the benefits of improving enrollee health status are apparent. Unfortunately, the financial benefits to the risk-bearing entity are somewhat diminished because of enrollee mobility. In other words, because of the often lengthy time delay between a large investment in early detection and prevention activities and the resulting cost savings to the system, individuals may have moved to other health plans and providers by the time there is a payoff.

There is plenty of anecdotal evidence to suggest that this phenomenon explains why most employers are leery of investing large amounts of money in safeguarding the health of their workforce, since the subjects of their investment may decide to switch jobs at any time. But the federal government knows that the Medicare program has the least transient patient population (once you qualify for Medicare, you are in for life), and as such is ideal for long-term health status improvement activities.

THE INFORMATION EXPLOSION AND THE EMPOWERED PATIENT

It has been suggested that forecasts about the future tend to overestimate the pace of change in the short run and underestimate it in the long run.

In late 1997, the Internet was the primary source of health information for only 2 percent of adult Americans. Television remained the primary source for 40 percent, and physicians were a close second at 36 percent.[9] But the growth of the Internet, as described elsewhere in this book, has been and will continue to be explosive.

One measure of this growth is the number of health-related documents identified on the World Wide Web by the AltaVista search engine. In January 1996, the keyword *health* resulted in approximately 800,000 hits, *medicine* resulted in 200,000, *pharmaceutical* resulted in 30,000, and *personal health* resulted in 1,000. By October 1998, the number of documents on the Web had climbed to 20.1 million for health, 5.2 million for medicine, 804,000 for pharmaceutical, and 23,800 for personal health.[10]

Self-Help Manuals

Idaho's Healthwise Communities project is a real-life case study in how providers can empower consumers to improve community health status and reduce costs at the same time. The goal of the project is to make some 280,000 residents of four Idaho counties the best informed, most empowered medical consumers possible. Spearheaded by Healthwise, Inc., a not-for-profit health education organization, the project began in early 1996 with the aid of a $2.1 million grant from the Robert Wood Johnson Foundation.

Working in concert with the major hospitals in the region and Blue Cross and Blue Shield of Idaho, some 125,000 *Healthwise Handbooks* were delivered to every residence in the four-county area. This user-friendly self-help manual describes nearly 200 common health problems, how an individual may treat the problem at home, and when a medical professional should be called. The book distribution was accompanied by a massive public awareness campaign, the establishment of a toll-free nurse help-line, an Internet site, and self-care resource centers located in libraries, hospitals, and worksites.

The results have been impressive. Six months after the book's release, 35 percent of the employee population stated that they had saved at least one doctor visit as a result.[11] Analysis of Blue Cross and Blue Shield of Idaho data further revealed that emergency room visits declined an average of 18 percent per customer.[12]

Communications Technology

B. C. Forbes of *Forbes* magazine once observed: "If you don't drive your business, you will be driven out of business." For hospital CEOs, the challenge of the future will not simply be to listen to the customer but to ensure that increasing patient activism is facilitated. Like it or not, patients will increasingly drive the business of health care, and hospitals must embrace this change. One way to accomplish this is through increased connectivity with patients; a critical mass of computer users will soon enable the widespread use of e-mail between physicians and patients. Computer technology plays a major role in this trend that will contribute to healthy communities and reduced utilization of health care resources.

Individuals who otherwise would have driven to the doctor's office or the emergency room to further examine a health problem can instead send an e-mail describing the symptoms and receive a written response from a physician. The development of remote sensor technology—such as glucose monitors, blood pressure cuffs, and immune assay kits—will allow the physician to access vital information about the patient remotely. At a minimum, the technology is now mature enough that every provider should consider incorporating some type of computer-based patient education into his or her practice.[13]

Although the federal government is likely to continue its vigilant regulation of telemedicine and medical software, communications technologies are evolving under substantially less scrutiny.[14] Aside from the obvious need to safeguard patient confidentiality, the provider field must also be mindful not to exacerbate the already acute problem of differential access to care among certain population groups. It stands to reason that low-income, lesser-educated individuals will be less likely to have a computer in their home and the knowledge to use it effectively to interact with medical professionals. Further, there are inherent dangers associated with the kind of unauthenticated information available on the Internet. There is a golden opportunity for academic medical centers to assume a leadership role in ensuring that patients and caregivers have access to accurate data online and that patient informatics becomes a core element in the training of new physicians.[15]

On the whole, emerging technologies will likely help, not hurt, disadvantaged populations. One specific example is the REMEC (Rural Emergency Medicine Education Consortium) system in Michigan's northern lower peninsula. Sponsored by a dozen hospitals in the region, the interactive video system provides educational programming, including EMT training and community health programs. In one case, a child from a low-income family experienced a gastrointestinal problem requiring treatment at the University of Michigan Medical Center in the southeast part of the state. Since follow-up visits there would have severely strained the family's financial resources, the UM specialists held six follow-up consultations via the REMEC network.[16]

From the hospital administrator's perspective, using physicians from outside the region through telemedicine creates a new headache: how to properly credential these providers and protect the institution from medical liability risk.

GIVING PATIENTS WHAT THEY WANT

At the same time that expensive, cutting-edge pharmaceuticals are increasingly being demanded by patients, the interest in alternative medicine is also skyrocketing.

Pharmaceuticals

Many health care firms, especially pharmaceutical makers, are taking advantage of the consumerism movement by dramatically stepping up their direct-marketing efforts to consumers. Aided by a liberalization of regulations by the Food and Drug Administration in 1997, expenditures for pharmaceutical advertising have skyrocketed from less than $100 million in 1990 to some $600 million today.[17] Combined with the ability to research the effectiveness of specific drugs and even join chronic disease chat rooms on the Internet where cutting-edge treatments are actively discussed, patients will increasingly demand certain prescriptions from their physicians.

Not surprisingly, pharmaceuticals are among the fastest growing components of the delivery system. In 1997, Blue Cross and Blue Shield of Michigan actually spent more money on pharmaceuticals ($423,006 per 1,000 subscribers) than it spent on inpatient hospital care ($381,893 per 1,000 subscribers) or physicians ($327,911 per 1,000 subscribers).[18]

There is now an intensifying debate on the overall impact of the introduction of expensive new drugs into the health care economy. The argument forwarded by the pharmaceutical industry is that drug use leads to reduced demand for surgical interventions and hospitalizations. No doubt this is true to a certain extent, and there can be no question that the introduction of some pharmaceuticals has improved quality of life and extended life expectancy. But taken as a whole, the net effect of these new pharmaceuticals is likely a significant increase in costs, since most of them—like most new technologies—are additive rather than substitutional. Many individuals who access new drugs would never have chosen invasive surgery that could have accomplished the same thing at higher expense. In other words, the prescription is not really saving money.

Such a phenomenon is not unprecedented in the annals of health policy. When a home health benefit was added to the Medicare program, the federal government expected to save money by virtue of the fact that for many beneficiaries, extremely expensive skilled nursing facility care would be replaced by the less expensive home care option. Instead, nursing home utilization continued to rise and a huge cohort of beneficiaries who had historically relied on family or friends to care for them in their own home (or simply chose to forgo any assistance) suddenly latched onto the new home care benefit. As a result, Medicare home health expenditures are projected to double by the year 2006, reaching $40 billion annually, without an accompanying reduction in nursing home costs.[19]

The Rise of Alternative Medicine

Alternative medicine, including homeopathy, naturopathy, reflexotherapy, aromatherapy, herbal medicine, and acupuncture, has been quite popular in other countries for many years. In Germany the national health insurance program provides coverage for a four- to six-week stay every three years at Kurkliniks, resort spas that provide mineral baths and other restorative treatments.[20]

In the United States, a recent study indicated that approximately 42 percent of the population uses some type of alternative care therapy.[21] Further, a survey of 125 U.S. medical schools revealed that nearly two-thirds are now teaching alternative medicine therapies.[22] For the most part, health plans have been making an effort to meet patients' wishes and add alternative medicine services to their list of covered benefits. This is a sound financial move to the extent that some individuals are intimidated by the formal medical delivery system and readily accept the far less expensive alternative therapy. But again, only time will tell whether the introduction of this new formalized benefit becomes a substitute or merely an addition to existing services. There is some evidence to suggest that it will be the latter, with only a tiny fraction of current alternative medicine users relying primarily on such treatments.[23]

TECHNOLOGY ADVANCES AND THE MANAGED CARE BACKLASH

Information technologies that assist patients in caring for themselves will be of enormous importance in the future. But there will always be a certain number of people who require treatment by medical professionals in a hospital or clinic setting. For this group, we have already seen significant improvements in medical technology, surgical techniques, and pharmaceutical development that have resulted in a radical shift to outpatient-based care. But in this respect we have come to a unique fork in the road, and it bears examination as we consider the increasing ability of technology to shorten hospital days and minimize contact with professional caregivers.

The bellwether case is the recent furor over maternity length of stay—identified by the media as "drive-through deliveries." Bills have surfaced in many states (and some have become law) that require HMOs to provide coverage to a mother and her newborn for a minimum period of inpatient hospital care (typically 48 hours following a natural birth, or 96 hours following a c-section). Many other procedures—like mastectomies—are targets of similar legislation.

In a time when the managed care industry has fallen into disfavor with the public, legislation of this type has instant appeal. It is no surprise that politicians have, for the most part, jumped on this bandwagon. However, there are some good reasons to be cautious as we proceed down this slippery slope.

First, any law that seeks to improve quality of health care should, at a minimum, be based on a thorough review of clinical outcomes (morbidity and mortality) data. It is not readily apparent that length-of-stay legislation is based on such a review, but the difficult factor to judge is the less tangible, but very real, psychological benefit that certain vulnerable patients experience simply from being in a hospital setting surrounded by capable professionals during a very anxious time in their lives. Other patients may feel more comfortable recovering in their own home, surrounded by familiar sights and sounds. The trouble with legislation is that it paints everyone with the same brush and could hinder physicians' ability to make appropriate choices based on their intimate knowledge of their patients. In any event, it is probably not the length of the hospitalization but rather the quality and quantity of education prior to a medical event and the extent of follow-up care after patients have returned to their home that determines the quality of the outcome.

The problem is that the lay public, fueled by the media, perceives that HMOs are endangering patients because they limit access to effective treatments in the name of cost control, and HMO physicians are not allowed to discuss the full range of treatment options for the same reason. In February 1997, Vice President Al Gore remarked that "[s]trict rules imposed by health plans have been turning the Hippocratic oath into a vow of silence." The perception is that managed care reimbursement methodologies create an incentive to *undertreat*.

Well known within the provider community, but less well known among the lay public, is the fact that traditional fee-for-service reimbursement creates incentives to *overtreat*. Any unnecessary medical intervention, whether it is invasive surgery or a drug prescription, creates the risk of an adverse outcome for the patient.

The challenge is to identify the *best* course of treatment for a given patient with a specific health problem. Advancements in computer science and information technology are beginning to give researchers the ability to analyze a massive volume of demographic, socioeconomic, and clinical outcomes data that will pave the way for the development of highly effective clinical pathways. As opposed to traditional pathways that were developed by a relatively small group of experts within a given specialty, pathways that are based on reams of scientific data will have a much better chance of gaining physician acceptance. In a recent nationwide survey of medical directors at HMOs, large group practices, and academic medical centers, fully 88 percent of respondents expected that a significantly larger share of clinical decisions will be covered by practice guidelines in five years.[24]

When this latter development occurs, an interesting phenomenon takes place. Physicians who believe in the power of effective pathways are much more willing to delegate patient care functions—particularly triaging—to nurses and physician assistants. This trend dovetails with the emphasis that managed care has placed on the development of care teams and, taken together, will likely narrow the gap between the information needs of physicians and midlevel providers.[25] The aforementioned survey of medical directors also identified that care teams will clearly be the preferred model for delivering services in the future, much more so than utilization of case managers, gatekeepers, or disease-state management companies.[26]

To health system administrators, this has enormous implications in terms of appropriate sizing of the medical staff and future partnership strategies with physicians. Over the past five years, hospitals and health systems have been aggressively acquiring physician practices. While this strategy is intended to safeguard patient referrals in the future, it has created a deluge of red ink in the present: the median hospital-owned physician practice is *losing* $46,577 per full-time-equivalent physician per year.[27]

The promise of information technology is to identify the most effective course of treatment, which obviously should result in cost savings over the long haul. But there could be another type of cost savings—if, in fact, clinical pathways allow more care to be delivered by midlevel practitioners, perhaps there will be less demand for the relatively higher-cost physicians.

The scope-of-practice issue is not new, but emerging technologies will clearly take us into the uncharted waters of this debate. Concomitantly, there is a growing consensus that physician supply may far exceed the U.S. demand in the very near future to such an extent that an American Medical Association spokesman recently stated that we could soon be in a position where "we will be eating our young."[28]

Y2K AND THE TECHNOLOGY BACKLASH

The discussion of Y2K—the year 2000 problem—that began among technophiles in the early 1990s has taken its place on center stage in the public consciousness. As the health care field begins to play catch-up with other industries that have invested proportionally more of their bottom lines in state-of-the-art information systems, the Y2K problem could not have come at a worse time.

The story of how this dilemma arose has been well documented. In short, the developers of the original legacy systems, with the assumed "19" in the year field, could not have imagined that the unwieldy model would, through constant adaptation, remain in use at the end of the millennium. The chaos resulting from old equipment that is not retooled to accept the year 2000 could potentially hit the health care field the hardest.

In addition to malfunctions in the systems that are common to all facilities (primary and emergency power generation, monitoring and security systems, fire alarms, elevators, and so on), hospital CEOs must also be prepared to deal with malfunctions in medical systems and equipment, including defibrillators, pacemakers, MRIs, CT scanners, and infusion pumps. Nurse call and telecommunications equipment, invoicing, shipping, license renewals, employee compensation and benefit administration, claims processing, and all manner of electronic data interchange are also in jeopardy. As a result of sorting and sequencing errors, schedules for clinic appointments, lab tests, admissions, and surgeries could be inexplicably rearranged, and patients' medical records and financial accounts could be rendered useless as well.[29]

If this scenario plays out, two key problems will develop. The first is an erosion of the confidence and trust of physicians in the hospital management, which will bear the blame for Y2K mishaps. This trust is especially critical as hospitals will increasingly attempt to partner with physicians in their community to form more tightly integrated financing and delivery vehicles. The second problem is the loss of consumer confidence in the health care system, particularly if there are adverse medical outcomes or a loss of patient confidentiality as a result of information system collapse.

THE FUTURE: TECHNOLOGY ENABLES HEALTHIER COMMUNITIES

Throughout this chapter, we have examined the forces driving change in the health care field, and the potential applications—and pitfalls—of computers and technology in the field. If we are successful at integrating the healthy communities model with the traditional medical model, it is very likely that emerging technologies will play a significant role.

As in many other industries, information is power in health care. The revolutionary advances in computer technology will give health care providers the ability to better assess the community's true health care needs, more effectively focus prevention and wellness programs, and improve the care of patients when they are admitted to the hospital.

References

1. InterStudy, National HMO Census Survey (1994).

2. U.S. Census Bureau, *Statistical Abstract* (Washington, DC: U.S. Government Printing Office, 1996).

3. Congressional Budget Office (1998), Web site www.cbo.gov.

4. HMO Performance Surveys, Group Health Association of America (1996, 1997).

5. Congressional Budget Office (1998), Web site www.cbo.gov.

6. Peters Seaman, "Do the Answers to U.S. Healthcare Problems Lie Within Canada?" *Michigan Hospitals* 27, no. 7 (August 1991): 21–27.

7. *Journal of Public Health Management and Practice* (March 1997).

8. Prospective Payment Assessment Commission, 1996 Annual Report to Congress.

9. Roper Starch Worldwide, Inc., survey for the National Health Council (fall 1997).

10. Institute for the Future, Conference on the Twenty-First Century Health Care Consumer, April 1998, unpublished research by Michigan Health & Hospital Association (October 1998).

11. Molly Metler and Donald W. Kemper, "In Support of Dr. Mom," *Healthcare Forum Journal* 40, no. 3 (May/June 1997): 60–63.

12. Colleen LaMay, "People Learning E.R. Means Emergency," *The Idaho Statesman* (January 22, 1998): 1C.

13. Murphy, "Computer-Based Patient Education," *Otolaryngological Clinician of North America* 31, no. 2 (April 1998): 309–17.

14. K. D. Mandl, I. S. Kohane, and A. M. Brandt, "Electronic Patient-Physician Communication: Problems and Promise," *Annals of Internal Medicine* 129, no. 6 (September 15, 1998): 495–500.

15. Braude Bader, "Patient Informatics: Creating New Partnerships in Medical Decision Making," *Academic Medicine* 73, no. 4 (April 1998): 408–11.

16. "Cyberstate.org," Michigan Information Technology Commission (September 1998), p. 27.

17. *Twenty-First Century Health Care Consumers* (Menlo Park, CA: Institute for the Future, 1998), p. 45.

18. *Blue Cross and Blue Shield of Michigan Fact Book* (1998).

19. Congressional Budget Office (January 1997).

20. Richard Knox, *Germany's Health System: One Nation, United With Healthcare for All* (New York: Faulkner & Gray, 1993), p. 50.

21. "The Landmark Report on Public Perceptions of Alternative Care," Landmark Healthcare, Inc. (1998).

22. M. S. Wetzel, D. M. Eisenberg, and T. J. Kaptchuk, "Courses Involving Complementary and Alternative Medicine at U.S. Medical Schools," *Journal of the American Medical Association* 280, no. 9 (September 2, 1998): 784–87.

23. John A. Astin, "Why Patients Use Alternative Medicine," *Journal of the American Medical Association* 279, no. 19 (May 20, 1998): 1548–53.

24. "A Look at the Future of Patient Care: A Survey of America's Medical Directors," Louis Harris and Associates, Inc. (July 1997).

25. Simpson: "The Role of Technology in Interdisciplinary Practice," *Nurse Manager* 29, no. 4 (April 1998): 20–22.

26. "A Look at the Future of Patient Care: A Survey of America's Medical Directors," Louis Harris and Associates, Inc. (July 1997).

27. Terese Hudson, "Necessary Losses?" *Hospitals and Health Networks* (December 20, 1997): 26.

28. Michael Scotti, MD, vice-president of medical education standards, American Medical Association (1997).

29. "Y2K: Mission Critical—An Executive Briefing for CEOs and Other Health Leaders," American Hospital Association (June 1998).

CHAPTER 11

A PAYER'S PERSPECTIVE ON THE FUTURE

Marianne Udow
Kevin L. Seitz

This chapter presents a more modest and cautious view on the impact of information technologies than the one presented by David Ellis. His vision of bots, quanta, nanotechnology, and MEMS is a far cry from our everyday world where success with automation is still measured largely by a payer's percentage of electronically transmitted claims. As a result, our opinions are formed by the constraints and the opportunities presented by information technology to an insurer who must continually balance cost and value in making business decisions aimed at achieving competitive advantages in the market. Unfortunately, to date much of the new technology has often been more hype than reality, offering potential for the future but less-than-advertised value added in the near term.

We also must confess to a bias, spurred by a predisposition regarding data and information technology. Stated simply, we believe it is misguided to assume that answers to fundamental questions can be gleaned from manipulating large data sets. The answers are not in the data but rather in our internal balancing of logic, common sense, compassion, ethics, and morality. Therefore, we are resistant to the idea that bots powered by artificial intelligence will ever replace physicians and others charged with directing care and making medical judgments. Instead, we see these technologies now and into the future as supports to the decision makers, helping them to diagnose and treat their patients using the most up-to-date and sophisticated techniques. This is fundamental to our vision of the future, for we see the physician-patient relationship continuing to exist as the basic building block for the health care system.

Our view is also more cautious because we use our past as a guide to the future. Looking back 20 years, medical care delivery and financing are essentially the same today as in 1979. Yes, there is more technology and less inpatient hospitalization, but changes in the delivery of care have not dramatically affected the functions of health insurers. These functions continue as integral components of the HMOs and the third-party administrators (TPAs) that have become more prominent in most markets. In addition, technology enhancements cannot be viewed in a vacuum. Other changes related to financing of health care, organization of medical care delivery, advances in medical science, and society's expectations regarding disease, aging, and quality of life will also have a fundamental impact on the functioning of insurers. Therefore, we see information technology as a key contributing factor but not a determining factor in defining the future role of the health insurance sector. Death, taxes, credit card interest, and group health insurance will likely be some of the inevitabilities that Americans continue to confront now and for at least the next 30 years.

Before we delve into the implications related to information and medical technology, we think it is important to highlight the potential structure of financing and its impact on the future of the insurance sector. The financial system for health care will have a major influence on defining service delivery and the methods of providing benefit coverage. This, in turn, will define the types of roles insurers can play. Within that structure, then, insurers will utilize technology to create competitive advantages.

HEALTH FINANCING

In the near term, we expect that the American health care system will remain largely employer financed, with the public sector plugging the gap through a categorical approach to covering needy populations. There may be tax credits, market reforms, patient bills of rights, or other statutory mandates, but the basic structure is likely to remain intact despite growing numbers of uninsured and continued escalation in costs.

Within this framework, there is one key financing trend that will fundamentally affect insurers; that is, employers will continue to move toward defined contribution approaches to financing group health coverages. A defined contribution is likely to become the preferred approach because an employer can set the amount it will pay and then the employee is free to choose among an array of coverage options. In effect, this shifts the actual purchasing responsibility from the employer to the employee, thereby converting group health insurance from a wholesale to a retail market. It also has the effect of shifting all or a portion of cost growth from the employer to the employee. Depending on one's ideology, this is either looked on as an innovative cost control mechanism or as simply a redistribution of cost to the individual.

In the retail world, consumers will want access to those providers that can best meet their needs. Consumerism will tend to disaggregate the delivery system into components, despite the continued consolidation of providers into integrated and quasi-integrated systems. This may evolve into a delivery structure where organized systems of care meet basic needs and outside/above these systems reside the specialties (the components) that consumers use as needed.

This trend toward consumer focus and "componentizing" providers will serve to reinforce many of the current functions of insurers. In particular, provider networking and customer service will be critical to insurer success. Other services, however, such as claims processing, will become less important as they can be readily provided by numerous entities. More important, in a retail market, insurers will be asked to provide value on an individual consumer basis. Later in this chapter, we will predict that this value will be created through data analysis to facilitate effective care management.

Ironically, the move to a retail market could in the long run prove to be the undoing of the current system of finance and the cozy niche occupied by most insurers. The American political system, based on the concept of interest group pluralism, weighs the competing/conflicting concerns of special interests in determining the public interest. The shift of purchasing responsibility to the individual will help create a very powerful special interest of consumers. We already see the influence of this group through the national movement for a patient bill of rights. This is likely a prelude to much more significant reform as consumers feel more and more of the cost burden associated with continued escalation in medical care expense. Defined contribution could be the spark for more fundamental reform, perhaps based on a hybrid of public tax-supported financing and managed competition among private plans. In this new world, the rules will truly change for insurers as they will be forced to compete based on their cost-effectiveness and ability to add value to a retail customer constituency, compared with the current world where the group purchaser is often the key decision maker. In this postreform world, there will be fewer winners, and they will be marked by their ability to harness information technology to their competitive advantage. In effect, fundamental health reform will make data analysis essential for the survival of insurers. The postreform winners will be distinguished by their provider networking and care management expertise.

With this structure and financing framework in mind, then, we think fundamental technology-driven change is likely. In the next section, we identify the major areas of technology change that are likely to affect payers. We then examine the implications of that change.

MAJOR TECHNOLOGY INNOVATIONS RELEVANT TO PAYERS

As noted by Ellis, technology innovations are expected to proceed in a broad range of areas that will affect every dimension of medical care, from patient encounter to diagnosis and treatment to administrative processing. From a payer's perspective, the major areas of impact are expected to include the following:

- Medical innovation
- Information transfer
- Back-end processing

Medical Innovation

Medical innovation includes the development of new technologies to treat disease, and anticipating new treatments will help payers predict cost trends. Technologies that are likely to result in a significant impact over the next 20 years include innovations on the genetic front for both diagnosis and treatment as well as the development of more sophisticated drug treatment regimens to treat a broad range of illnesses, especially those most likely to afflict an aging population.

Over just the past several years, we have seen tremendous innovation in medical technology. New diagnostic procedures have enabled a more precise determination of patient care needs. In addition, new drug therapies are enabling more people to live longer, more productive lives. And new, less invasive surgical procedures are allowing more individuals to receive treatment, whereas in the past the risks of the treatment may have outweighed the potential benefits.

For the most part, this new technology has raised health care costs, and that trend is expected to continue into at least the near future. For example, the cost of drugs per Blue Cross and Blue Shield of Michigan member in 1998 increased almost 15 percent and is expected to grow at a similar rate in 1999. This increase is due to a combination of factors, including the development of new and better drugs as well as more individuals being provided drugs for more indications.

Microinvasive procedures such as laparoscopy have already increased the number of potential patients for procedures, whereas in the past the risks of the procedure would have likely outweighed the potential benefits in many cases. Already, for example, new, minimally invasive heart bypass surgery is in the experimental stage. Should such a procedure be determined to be safe and effective, many heart patients now maintained through drug regimens are likely to turn to surgery more quickly. Such surgical procedures, though costing less than current surgical procedures, cost more than alternate treatment regimens. Thus, overall health care costs can be expected to increase.

Finally, genetic technology is on the verge of making a major impact on health care through early diagnosis of a broad range of conditions, resulting in much earlier intervention (even to the point of correcting some genetic problems during pregnancy). It took 50 years of basic human genome research to gain the knowledge that bacteria were responsible for diseases such as pneumonia. Treatment with sulfa drugs followed, with tremendous impact on the rates of fatal pneumonia in the population. The Human Genome Project has followed a similar trajectory and is coming close to the point where the basic research is likely to produce substantive new treatments. Indeed, a team of 64 scientists from the National Institutes of Health and the British Sanger Center have just been able to produce a new "gene map" that pinpoints the chromosomal locations for nearly half of all genes.[1] This new map charts the chromosomal locations of 30,181 human genes, and the accuracy of that mapping has been improved two to three times compared with the earlier version. The map provides a scientific infrastructure for understanding how genes interact with one another to maintain normal health and how defects can lead to illnesses such as cancer and heart disease. This achievement is expected to help expedite the development of treatments for cancer, hypertension, mental illness, and other genetically linked diseases.

Information Transfer

Health plan identification cards today are far more basic than many credit cards in active use. Today, these cards simply contain information on health benefit plan coverages and transmit basic billing instructions to health plans. The introduction of smart cards carrying both clinical and administrative information has been discussed in the health care field for more than 10 years. For a variety of reasons, this type of card has not been pursued to any large degree. These reasons include the fact that the initial investment to develop the cards is very high and the technology to use them is not readily available. In addition, because today most health plans use their own billing and coding conventions, there is little transferability of the cards and the data they contain among plans, providers, consumers, and employers.

However, to the extent that a national database and patient identifier proves to be a politically viable path in the next 5 to 10 years, the likelihood of a smart card will increase. This card will provide a much more accessible source of data for payers, physicians, and other providers of care. It will increase the portability of health care coverage as well as making information transfer to payers a more direct, timely, and lower-cost process. Indeed, through this mechanism, payers and providers will have access to critical clinical information as well as the basic claims-type information available today.

Back-End Processing

Today, health plans are pleased when they are able to increase their electronic billing percentages. Many claims of many payers continue to be handled with extensive paper submissions. An increase in electronic billing can reduce the cost of claims processing per claim by more than half because human interaction is reduced. An electronic billing rate of 80 percent is considered high. Indeed, estimates are that only 62 percent of claims will have been submitted electronically in 1998.[2] Although this represents an increase from prior years, it is still quite low and paper continues to be quite common. Predictions are being made today that the availability of the Internet will fundamentally change the payment system for providers. The increasing use, sophistication, and security of the Internet system will enable more direct data transfer and essentially eliminate the need for claim forms and the like. In combination with the smart card and new banking alternatives, direct information and financial transfers can occur. In addition, consumers will have access to their own health care information and status of their health benefits and coverage through electronic mechanisms.

IMPLICATIONS FOR INSURERS

It is important to put these medical, information, and payment technologies into perspective to more precisely estimate their impact on insurers. Cautions include the following:

- Many health plans will be slow to fully exploit use of new technology. In addition, most of the uninsured will not have access to more sophisticated and costly medical treatments. As a result, providers will need to maintain parallel systems to accommodate insurers and patients who continue to interact on a mostly manual, encounter-by-encounter basis.
- Structural and cultural systems are slower to change than are technological systems. For example, we do not agree with the premise that doctors' offices will become virtual offices. We believe that patients will still want to see their doctors in some form. Even in the most fanciful *Star Trek* theories of medical care, the care itself is still delivered by a caring physician, vastly aided by diagnostic and therapeutic technology. Care will certainly be aided—but not replaced—by technology.
- Key functions that insurers perform today are likely to continue in some form; though other entities besides what we know as payers today are likely to be able to perform many of the functions now done principally by health care payers.
- Last, but by no means least, no one can actually predict the future because there are so many contingencies and unforeseen events that will influence trends that look likely to come to pass.

Thus, much of what we say here may turn out to be completely erroneous. However, there are some trends that are developing with regard to technology that seem quite plausible, and it is worthwhile to understand and plan for these kinds of trends. Our focus is on some of these plausible scenarios.

Given all of the caveats noted above, then, what are some of the plausible scenarios and implications for health care insurers? There are three general predictions that we would like to focus on specifically:

1. Many critical functions that insurers perform and compete over today are likely to be commoditized and automated.
2. Intermediaries will continue to exist in some form, but their functions will shift from an emphasis on administration (claims processing and the like) to an emphasis on data analysis leading to more sophisticated approaches to care management.
3. The cost of medical care is a wild card in this picture: technology has the potential to both cause substantial savings in medical costs and increase those costs. Depending on the course that's followed, fundamental changes for payers are likely as a result of medical innovations.

Commoditization of Key Functions

Historically, the key functions of insurers have been underwriting, rating, sales, benefit and product design, customer servicing, claims administration, provider contracting, and use and quality management. Some of these functions are likely to be much less significant in the future than they are today. For example, medical underwriting has been reduced as a result of the Health Insurance Portability and Accountability Act (HIPAA) of 1996. Over the next several years, it is likely that further legislative change will be made to reduce this administrative function within insurance even more.

Predicting cost trends to establish appropriate pricing, on the other hand, is likely to stay a major function of insurers and will probably continue to be as much an art as a science. Though genetic testing has the potential to identify likely health problems for individuals, federal and state legislation will most certainly keep this information confidential and not usable by health care (or other) insurers. Thus, accurate predictors of an individual's future health profile will continue to remain elusive. Without this information, establishing future rate trends to enable pricing of health benefits is likely to continue to rely principally on historical trends adjusted for new medical care treatments expected to come online in the coming year. Thus, though new data systems may enable more complex assessments of cost profiles of individuals, in the end both epidemiological information and the technology innovations will remain difficult to predict, requiring rating systems that rely on judgment as well as analysis.

The sales, benefit and product design, and customer servicing functions may be significantly changed through technology that is likely to be available in the near term. Indeed, especially with the advent of the Internet, many purchaser and consumer transactions that now take place in person or on the phone can take place in an online mode. In addition, the technology that is enabled by smart cards (described below and in chapter 3), can significantly aid the sales effort by providing enhanced data-tracking tools identifying in detail the nature of those consumers who stay and those that leave a health insurer. Thus, retention rates can be analyzed with more precision and products adjusted much more quickly to meet purchaser and consumer goals.

These changes in regard to sales and customer service will require a fundamentally different insurer workforce. Today, consumer contact with health plans is generally fairly limited. Most consumers receive some written communications from health plans, including their identification card with basic information on their scope of coverage, Explanation of Benefit forms when the consumer uses health services, and periodic newsletters providing general health information. In addition, customer service representatives provide answers to inquiries on problems with or questions about health benefits. Relatively few people are needed to prepare the written materials and most inquiries are handled by telephone. Phone inquiries use computer-assisted systems that track benefits and claims payment for an individual member.

With advances in artificial intelligence, it is anticipated that voice response systems and online communications modalities will be used to respond with increasing degrees of complexity and sophistication. As Internet usage increases, written communication is likely to be more prevalent and instantaneous responses the norm. Health insurer Web sites are already beginning to provide provider directory information, basic health care information, and general health plan information (such as phone numbers and addresses). In the future, these sites are likely to provide even more health information as well as offering an interactive forum for communication. For many carriers, the Internet may well be the primary site for answering inquiries of both consumers and providers.

Thus, though most of the administrative technology described in this chapter reduces human intervention, Internet communication technology can actually increase human involvement and requires a higher skill level than is generally in place today. In order to handle the Internet communications and ensure both accuracy and clarity of responses, customer service representatives will need to have much more sophisticated written communication skills as well as needing to be technology literate to a greater degree than they are today. This demand for a smaller but more highly skilled workforce has many profound implications that will directly affect health insurers' location decisions and hiring practices. For example, because of technology, the health insurance workforce may become global, less reliant on local communities for customer service workers. Many high schools in this country are not preparing their students for work in a technologically enhanced environment that places an increasing emphasis on written communication skills. Thus, communities that have relied on these kinds of health care jobs are likely to find fewer of their citizens employed unless they are preparing now for this new future.

Claims administration is also likely to be fundamentally changed. As noted earlier, for many insurers claims administration currently involves a considerable amount of paper. Indeed, technological innovation in this regard has slowed somewhat over the past several years as payers, billers, providers, and the government have committed substantial resources to solving the year 2000 computer problem. It is likely that even after the turn of the century, there will be many health plans, including, apparently, the federal government, that will be continuing to devote resources to correcting basic functioning within their computer systems.

Ten years or so in the future, however, claims administration is almost certain to be fully automated. This automation is likely to be facilitated by public policy decisions that will make transportability more feasible. Today, there is considerable variation between plans and states with regard to billing codes, identification numbers, and other processing conventions. HIPAA includes a provision on administrative simplification intended to reduce this complexity.

HIPAA does not mandate electronic data interchange, but it does require the use of standard formats, code sets, and identifiers for those plans that do transact information electronically. Today, there are no billing clearinghouses that can handle all HIPAA-required transactions in the mandated 4010 version of standards from the American National Standards Institute Accreditation Committee.[3] Thus, claims clearinghouses and others will be devoting considerable resources to modifying their systems over the next few years to be able to accept these billing formats.

HIPAA also contemplates a universal identification number that would permit central storage of data and access to these data for health services research purposes. That concept has come under significant attack because of concerns about patient confidentiality. However, it is most likely that over the next five to ten years, many of the variations in billing and coding practices will be substantially reduced even if the uniform identification number does not get implemented.

Billing-type services will continue to be needed, but information and financial transfers will probably be instantaneous, as will the transmittal of critical medical care information.

Smart cards, too, have the potential to substantially change the administrative functions performed by insurers. Smart cards will enable physicians to receive real-time eligibility, precertification or authorization, drug interaction information, and formulary information, among other things. From the payers' perspective, in addition to helping with claims interaction, these cards can help simplify the enrollment process and improve the accuracy of data once they are uniformly available because such information will be transferable from one payer to another. In addition, by transmitting critical health management information to providers, these cards can help improve the management of health care costs. Finally, smart cards will also enable patients to monitor the status of their claims and their own medical records and even make their next appointments.

Smart cards can significantly improve the efficiency of the health care administrative process. Comparing these cards with bank ATM cards illustrates the efficiency potential. In this regard, banks have reported lowering their costs per transaction from $1.08 to 13 cents.[4]

With uniform billing forms and coding systems, insurers will not, in any significant way, distinguish themselves based on the variations they can create to manage cost through benefit administration. Rather, these services will be commoditized and performed by the lowest-cost vendors, which may or may not include the current health care insurers.

Provider contracting will continue to be a key function of inter-mediaries. Whether or not it is an insurer, an employer, government, or another independent entity, the ability to put together high-quality, accessible networks of physicians and other caregivers will be a neces-sary service on behalf of consumers. In effect, in this model, insurers that can be "integrators" of networks of providers will have a distinct advantage. Indeed, with the information provided through smart cards, health care payers will have much more useful information to use to develop high-quality provider networks. In addition, information on the provider network, including appointment-scheduling options, can be made readily available to consumers through the insurers themselves.

Use and care management practices performed by health insurers are also likely to go through a substantial transformation due to emerg-ing technology. Today, use management systems rely on statistical mod-els that attempt to predict provider behavior so that audits can be focused on the most likely candidates for inappropriate billing practices. In addition, these systems use historical claims data to identify potential procedures of concern or to profile providers and share with them infor-mation about their use patterns that may look inconsistent with that of their peers. These systems also use rudimentary claims information to identify and work with patients who are now using considerable health resources or who are expected to do so in the near future.

All of these practices attempt to improve the cost-effectiveness of the health care delivery system. However, the effectiveness of these systems is seriously limited by time lags in the receipt of critical data necessary to identify the patient, physician, or procedure where a special focus is appropriate. They also lack the comprehensiveness necessary for accu-rately and effectively establishing an appropriate focus and intervention plan. Claims information often has a 60-day or longer lag time from the date of service because of delays in billing and reporting systems. There-fore, many of the action steps taken are based on old information, and problems may well grow in the absence of timely action.

In the future the information available in this regard will be much broader and more accessible, and the timeliness of the data will be enor-mously enhanced. With smart cards, information transfer should be vir-tually instantaneous. In addition, this information will include key clinical information that goes far beyond the billing data available today. With this information, health care insurers (or others) can be more pre-cise in establishing appropriate areas of focus and can intervene quickly if necessary before patient treatment has progressed to a significant degree. Finally, the intervention can be much more thoughtful and analytically sound in that it will be based on a breadth of information that includes clinical indicators now only available through medical chart review. These enhancements will affect all use, care, and disease management programs.

This information availability also has tremendous staffing implications for health care payers. Again, data availability will reduce the need for staff who currently spend considerable time auditing medical records. On the other hand, as with the need for a different customer service workforce, the availability of more clinically sophisticated data will require a different type of worker able to analyze the extensive information that is provided and work closely in partnership with both providers and consumers of care.

New Emphases

Health insurers today compete on the basis of their low cost. They achieve their competitive advantage largely through efficient, effective claims processing, discounts from provider contracts, ability to reduce inpatient hospital days, and, unfortunately, risk selection. In the future, though health insurers will continue to compete based on cost, the elements of competitive advantages will be quite different. Successful intermediaries will be those that are able to manage vast stores of data, working with both consumers and providers of care to help them navigate the health care system as well as manage the cost and quality of care. Health intermediaries may well stitch together the commodity products of claims processing, rating, and the like. But the core functions will be the transmittal and analysis of data and the provision of consumer services.

Consumer Education and Information. Because, as noted in the health finance section, health care is likely to increasingly shift from a wholesale to a retail market over this period, intermediaries will communicate more directly with the consumer than they do today. The increase in medical technology noted above is likely to present consumers with more choices and more potential confusion as they try to sort out the appropriate care path and caregiver. Intermediaries can provide consumers with a valuable service if they can become a central source of consumer education and information about treatment modalities and provider options. By maintaining and sharing large databases, intermediaries can make available outcomes data on large population groups that will enable consumers to make better choices about their own health care. The connection between health care carriers and consumers, then, in this vision of the future, will become direct and personal. The consumer will be able to rely on the insurer as a navigator of the system as well as a source for clinically sound information—a centralized location for health services research and outcomes data on both procedures and providers of care.

In order for this role to become a realistic one for a health care insurer, many insurers will have to change their basic approach to insurance coverage. That is, over the past 30 years or so, most insurers have attempted to make profits through selection of low-risk individuals rather than by providing true care management. Although this practice has been limited by HIPAA, many health insurers continue risk selection in more subtle ways. Risk avoidance and other factors associated with an employer-financed system have led many consumers to view insurers with suspicion and have, indeed, resulted in many cases where consumers and insurers are operating at cross-purposes.

Given a 20-year time horizon, however, it is possible that some form of (at least) national health policy will develop that will reduce the role of health insurers in benefit design and truly eliminate practices that reward insurers for risk selection rather than care management. If such a transformation occurs, the insurers' role can be fundamentally altered into that of a critical source for consumer education and information. In this context, then, in the future the term *intermediary* might be better than *health insurer* or *health plan*. This concept of mediator or go-between between the patient and the health care system will be tremendously important in the increasingly complex health care system of the future.

Health Services Research and Provider Data Management. Connected to the concept of consumer intermediary is the role of data manager. It is the access to clinically meaningful data about both providers and clinical care that enables health insurers to become consumer intermediaries. Access to the data also enables insurers to provide critical information for research directed at improving health care delivery and quality. With the availability of clinical data, then, intermediaries can work with physicians and other researchers to study outcomes, perform epidemiological analyses, and the like to better understand the impact of different treatment strategies.

In addition, these data can be of enormous value to providers of care in enabling them to improve their practice. Intermediaries can more precisely monitor provider behavior and intervene quickly through network selection, education, breakthrough processes, and other approaches to share information to educate and improve the consistency and quality of care. Through sharing of this information with both the public and providers of care, the costs of clinical care can be better managed and the outcomes and quality of care can be continually enhanced. This intermediary role can be independent of the role of consumer intermediary and, by itself, can be a major focus and value added for health care insurers for the future.

Medical Care Costs

The wild card in all of this discussion about the role of health care payers in the future is the issue of the costs of medical care. No one can know for certain what will happen in the next 20 years with regard to medical technology. However, regardless of what happens, medical care cost trends will have a major impact on the role of health insurers. In 1992, the double-digit increases in medical care led many in the middle class to fear that they were likely to lose their health insurance coverage. In the end, the proposals put forward by the Clinton administration raised more concerns among interest groups than the status quo, and so health care reform failed. Since that time, health care cost increases have moderated considerably. However, there are signs that costs are again on the rise. Indeed, the Health Care Financing Administration just released a study that predicts a doubling of health care costs by the year 2007.[5] If cost escalation returns to the levels of the early '90s, it is likely there will be another wave of interest in fundamental health care reform. Such an eventuality could substantially change the role (if any) of health care insurers in the future. Thus, medical care costs could have the greatest impact of any future trend on the predictions that we have made to date.

The future of medical care costs is far from certain, but the two ends of the spectrum can be predicted. On one end, medical technology could develop in such a way that care strategies become so effective that the approximately 25 major diseases in the developed world are eliminated. In that scenario, we would have what Lewis Thomas called "the genuinely decisive technology of modern medicine." This kind of "full-blown" technology understands the underlying mechanism of a disease so that relatively inexpensive and simple things can halt it (the polio vaccine is an example of full-blown technology). At the other end of the spectrum, we could continue with "halfway" technologies—which is what most technology enhancements are producing today—in which medical care deals with just the results of the illness without understanding its underlying mechanism.[6]

In the full-blown technology end of the spectrum, health care costs could actually be substantially reduced. While death would not be avoided, it would be a collapse of all systems without being preceded by the chronic diseases common today.[7] At the other end of the spectrum, halfway technology will almost certainly increase costs because we are likely as individuals to live longer and with more chronic conditions. This means that though there may be an increase in productivity and contribution to society at large because of increased longevity, medical care costs themselves would be most likely to increase substantially.

The full-blown technology scenario is not as far-fetched as it may seem. Indeed, that is exactly the intent and direction of the Human Genome Project. As noted above, human gene research has been under way for almost 50 years now and is on the verge of major breakthroughs in the full mapping of the chromosomal locations of all genes. When this work is completed, enormous breakthroughs should be possible in detection and treatment of common illnesses. Lewis Thomas believes that for every disease there is a "single key mechanism that dominates all others." If this mechanism can be found, then the disorder itself can be controlled. He predicted in the 1970s that the major diseases of human beings are an "approachable biological puzzle . . . [that is] ultimately solvable."[8] Lewis Thomas's predictions are as fresh today as they were in the 1970s, and the Human Genome Project seems poised to justify his optimistic assessment of our ability to expand the extent of our full-blown technology.

Of course, over the next 20 years the true picture is most probably going to be somewhere between those two ends of the spectrum. That is, it is likely that full-blown technology will increase and we will indeed be able to cure things in the future that are chronic conditions today (such as rheumatoid arthritis) or prevent rather than delay such diseases as heart disease, cancers, and stroke. At the same time, however, we are likely to continue to develop halfway technologies that will not only improve the quality of life and reduce morbidity but also increase the cost of medical care. For example, the new drugs entering the market in 1999 are almost all halfway technologies. New treatments for arthritis (the Cox 2 Inhibitors), mental illness, obesity, and the like reduce the symptoms without eliminating the disease. Tamoxifen may be a first step at prevention of breast cancer, but the research is uncertain in this regard and Tamoxifen cannot be touted as preventing breast cancer but, rather, as potentially delaying the onset of the disease. In addition, the potential side effects are significant enough that many women will not want to pursue this course of treatment. New treatments in the pipeline are indeed expected to improve the quality of life of some individuals, but they will also almost certainly increase the cost of care.

To the extent that the next several years produce a mix of full-blown and halfway technologies, the pressure on health insurers to limit the scope of what is covered is likely to grow enormously. That pressure has already been evident with Viagra, the impotence-reducing drug. Kaiser Permanente determined (until regulatory authorities intervened) that it would not cover Viagra simply on the grounds that the cost outweighed its potential benefits. This kind of debate and dialogue are likely to increase over at least the next five years or so. To the extent, then, that consumers, especially the middle class, believe that they are not being provided with the medical care that they need and deserve, the political pressure for change in the health care system will grow. However, even if government does indeed step into the picture and we develop a more centralized administrative process much like the rest of the developed world, the impact of technology noted in the previous sections will still be relevant. That is, the administrative enhancements that will reduce the cost of key insurance functions will occur under whatever model of health care is in place, as will online, real-time availability of clinically meaningful data. What is less clear is the likelihood that the consumer intermediary model and the data research model would develop in a fundamentally different health care system than we have today. Those scenarios could vary substantially depending on the nature of the health care system in place in the future.

Whatever the future brings, then, with regard to technology's impact on the administrative functions of health care insurers, its impact on medical care itself is likely to dwarf all of the other changes. The future in this regard is both exciting to consider and daunting to envision.

CAUTIONS AND CONCLUSIONS

In table 11-1, we have attempted to summarize the previous discussion and display how we see insurer functionality changing in response to technology advances over the next several years. The table distinguishes between the near-term and long-term state of the industry. This distinction is important, for in the near term, insurers will be involved in retooling themselves to create online, interactive capabilities and set the stage for their new role as data integrators. In the longer term, technology should allow a melding of insurer and provider functions into a single process at the point of care, in which the provider and the patient receive instantaneous feedback on treatment options, best practices, and benefit plan coverages and payments.

It is important to note that technology is expensive. It will require large capital investments by insurers, and they will expect a clear-cut rate of return. Given the uncertain value of new technology, many insurers will proceed with caution, allowing others to take the risks and break new ground. As a result, it is likely that actual change will occur more slowly than knowledge about, and our capability to adopt, new technologies. It is likely that much of this technology will remain proprietary in the short run, serving as a competitive advantage for the few who decide to risk their traditional roles for the potential of generating value in their new roles as integrators. This is a major reason why our near-term vision is actually quite modest. We believe that it could take several years for new technology to be converted from a private good to a social good.

A further caution is warranted based on an observation regarding how medicine is practiced by most physicians. Physicians today function very much in a production environment. Their time is parceled into 15-minute segments, and many tasks are repetitive and impractical for translation into databases. Therefore, there will always be a challenge to develop data sets that allow for comprehensive and actionable assessments of quality. Generally speaking, if data are not linked to monetary payment, then they are unreliable and not worth the cost of collection. Even with the link to payment, data integrity remains an obstacle to full realization of the change potential presented by emerging technologies.

Despite these cautions, we see a changing world for insurers. Unless health care experiences fundamental financial reform (inspired by consumers and cost escalation), it is most likely that insurers will still be very much a part of the health care system 30 years from now. Their functions will change, but not to the extent that they are unrecognizable

Table 11-1

INSURER FUNCTIONALITY		
	Current State of the Industry	Near-Term State	Long-Term State
Claims Processing	Mix of paper and electronic claims; systems converting to online adjudication; providers supplied with group eligibility and coverages through online systems	Elimination of paper; provider ability to track pending claims online; provision of patient history to providers online (from single insurer)	Claims adjudication at point of care and integrated with caregiving process; patient history across payers available as public good
Rating and Underwriting	Time-lagged, dated claims data used; process imprecise; Industry prone to underwriting cycles	Data more timely due to online claims processing; continued reliance on claims data; smoothing of underwriting cycles; still more art than science	Instantaneous data; under-writing function probably shifted to public sector; rating now split evenly between art and science
Customer Service	Phone prompts and voice message systems for basic plan information; customer service reps (CSR) handle routing and complex inquiries; limited ability to fully resolve issue at point of inquiry	Internet used to enhance CSR interface; value-added retail services, such as appointment scheduling and online physician prescribing; online CSR capability to fully resolve inquiries	Automated inquiry resolution enhanced through voice response and artificial intelligence advances; CSRs required as skilled troubleshooters

(Continued on next page)

Table 11-1 (Continued)

INSURER FUNCTIONALITY		
	Current State of the Industry	**Near-Term State**	**Long-Term State**
Provider Network Management	Networks distinguished by discounts and access; quality assured through credentialing that relies on professional certifications; claims-based profiling and peer review	Networks continue to be distinguished by discounts and access; designation of providers that meet quality and specialty standards based on risk-adjusted outcomes data; timely and focused data for profiling; reliable risk adjustment systems and quality benchmark standards	Networks continue to be distinguished by discounts and access; integration of medical record with insurer-paid claims; provides robust basis for quality analysis; comparative reliable information on providers available in public domain
Use Management	Rudimentary analysis of outdated paid claims to target areas for intervention; precertification of high-cost cases; reliance on retrospective medical record reviews for recovery actions	More timely and focused data analysis; opportunities for intervention during care process in limited situations; delegation of use management functions to high-performing provider groups	Integration of claims adjudication and best-practices assessment at point of care providing instantaneous feedback on appropriateness of planned treatment

Table 11-1 (Continued)

INSURER FUNCTIONALITY		
	Current State of the Industry	**Near-Term State**	**Long-Term State**
Care Management	Development of high-cost case management as core plan function; experimentation with unproven disease management programs	Development of predictive models regarding who would benefit from disease management; validation of value of mid-range disease management	Care management and use management coverage at point of care through instantaneous feedback
Sales	Reliant on personal relationships, sales reps, market preset packages of benefits	Reliant on personal relationships, ability to customize benefits and rate them at point of sale	Reliant on personal relationships, ability to integrate claims and other data to develop retention strategy

from their 1999 versions. Insurers will continue to define themselves based on their ability to network with providers and mediate the process that transfers dollars from consumers to providers. But the value equation will change in that insurers will distinguish themselves from their competitors by their ability to analyze data and use this information to support providers in the provision of care. Table 11-2 summarizes this shift in areas of competitive advantage that will gradually occur within the health insurance sector.

Also, it is important to remember our wild card. Advances in medical technology could drastically change the above scenarios; that is, substantial increases in medical costs could result in fundamental system reforms that move us closer to a single-payer system.

Complex problems rarely have simple solutions. Similarly, the complexities of the insurance business will not translate into a single prototype for the insurer of the future. Different plans will emphasize different core competencies. But larger carriers will need to demonstrate value in

Table 11-2

CHANGING ROLE OF INSURERS	
Current State	**Future State**
Competition based on low cost	Competition based on low cost and consumer support
Competitive advantage achieved through: • claims processing • provider discounts • risk selection • benefit cost management • customer service (problem resolution)	Competitive advantage achieved through: • data management to facilitate care management • personal connection with consumer • provider network management • stitching of commodity functions

the management of health care costs, and it would appear that this road is paved with the new technologies that will facilitate their maturation as data integrators. Interestingly, this does appear to raise questions regarding the future viability of gatekeeper managed care products, but that is best left for another chapter in another book.

References

1. "Human Genome Project Reaches a Milestone," *Healthcare Weekly Review* 14, no. 32 (1998): 3.

2. Alice McCart, ed., *Health Data Directory, 1997* (New York: Faulkner & Gray, 1996), p. 5.

3. Ibid.

4. Raymond J. Hennessey, "Smart Cards Are in the Pipeline," *Best's Review* 99, no. 1, supplement (1998): 27.

5. Sheila Smith et al., "The Next Ten Years of Health Spending: What Does the Future Hold?" *Health Affairs* 17, no. 5 (1998): 128–40.

6. Lewis Thomas, *The Lives of a Cell: Notes of a Biology Watcher* (New York: Viking Penguin, 1978), pp. 32, 34.

7. Lewis Thomas, *The Medusa & the Snail: More Notes of a Biology Watcher* (New York: Viking Penguin, 1995), p. 141.

8. Ibid., pp. 140–41.

CHAPTER 12

LEADERSHIP, FOLLOWERSHIP, AND SCIENCE

Craig Ruff

Mr. Parker, do you know what it means to feel like God?
—*Island of Lost Souls*, Erle C. Kenton, Paramount, 1933, based on the H. G. Wells novel *The Island of Dr. Moreau*

Fasten your seat belts, it's going to be a bumpy night.
—*All About Eve*, Joseph L. Mankiewicz, 20th Century-Fox, 1950

The world has entered the golden age of biology. Assumptions about human health are unraveling, consumer expectations are skyrocketing, and health care leaders are assuming God-like powers.

The next quarter-century will be bumpy. Scientific fact will strain humans' ability to keep pace. In equal measure, biology will extend benefits to, and challenge, life. People will live longer and learn faster. Can society and nature afford the benefits? Can we handle the stress? Can we remodel organizations to adjust? Can we maintain egalitarian ideals and altruistic mission? The thorny questions that science poses will not be answered by scientists. They will be answered by leaders like you.

For 250,000 years of human life on Earth, each age has foisted on leaders opportunities and problems. A society as small as a family or as large as a nation craves leadership to differentiate itself from others, defend life and possessions, form and bring about adherence to values, and persevere until tomorrow.

Had you lived in an earlier age, you could have been a leader of a family of hunter-gatherers, a nomadic tribe, an army of barbarians, a walled city, a nation, or an empire. Fate dealt you the hand of leading today: not a nation, but a community. Not soldiers, but the sick. Not a government, but a health care system.

You will spend only a flicker of time leading human progress on this planet, but know this: no leader coming before you ever had the power to influence the future that you hold. To instill a bit of humility, know that every leader to come will have even greater power.

AXIOMS

This chapter is about health care leadership in an age of scientific advance. The axioms of this essay are pretty straightforward:

- Health care leaders do not have to be scientists, but they need to know enough about science to be helpful, maybe even dangerous at times, to science.
- Health care leaders must engage, earn, and hold the trust of followers—the general public. Many in the tribe—your community's residents—will be befuddled by science and need your caring and deliberative guidance.
- Followers must want to be informed, hold leaders accountable, and know when to change them. Leaders can help them on all these fronts.
- Scientists do not have to be leaders, but they need to weigh the consequences of their inventions on leaders and followers.

A healthy community—one that is enlightened—is one in which leadership, "followership," and science mesh. In that healthy community the following conditions hold:

- People expect medical help to be affordable.
- Miracles are fairly meted out.
- Consequences on aspects of life other than health are weighed.
- Research findings in Geneva or Atlanta are delivered *just in time* to your hometown, but community research plays a compelling role, too.
- Politics mediates faith and science and is respected and trusted to do so.

- Leaders are patient with followers, accepting their false assumptions, desire for quick fixes, judgmental instincts, and greed.

You may be a hospital trustee, an auxiliary volunteer, a physician, nurse, or other clinician, a fundraiser, a philanthropist, or an administrator. What you are is a health care leader. Bumpy as the times may be, just know that what decisions you make, how you make them, and how you communicate them make a difference in your community. Because you may not get all the thanks you deserve, I thank you for caring.

BURDENS OF LEADERS

Leadership done well carries a price. It means that you change the course of society, and people would live differently were it not for you. They may be better off or worse off. Leaders first do no harm. Great leaders then do good. You—a leader—play God with lives. That ought to be the first line in your job description, inherent in your roles and responsibilities as a health care leader. Being a follower carries a price, too. Followers must separate the wheat from the chaff offered by leaders. They must trust but verify, as the Russian proverb advises.

Science and technology have raised the ante dramatically in health care leadership and followership. Tomorrow, the stakes are limitless for longevity and quality of life. With every medical miracle, responsibilities pile upon one another, building a tower of influence, power, expectations, and vulnerability.

Relations with Science

With few exceptions, leaders in American hospitals, churches, synagogues, philanthropic organizations, economic clubs, capitols, and companies are not scientists. They are blissfully unaware of science. When was the last time that your Rotary, Lions, or Zonta club scheduled as speaker a scientist, as opposed to a political, business, philanthropic, or labor leader or poet, composer, or historian? CEOs will shell out a thousand bucks for a seminar on Eternal Quality Management through Endless Enhancement, but surf past a half-hour Discovery Channel program on biodiversity.

Our politicians—to single out one leadership cadre—are lawyers, city planners, Realtors, insurance agents, retailers, stockbrokers, residential builders, farmers, factory workers, police officers, clergy, school coaches, accountants, sociologists, public relations experts, journalists, marketers, manufacturers, and economists. Occasionally, a physician, engineer, psychologist, or math or science teacher becomes an officeholder, but that is pretty rare. Rarer still does electoral politics attract a nuclear physicist such as Michigan Congressman Vernon Ehlers or a marine biologist such as the former governor of Washington Dixie Lee Ray.

Mind you, nobody wants a state legislature or city hall inhabited only by scientists. Government is not a laboratory, and citizens are not frogs. But good leaders, including those in governance, engage in followership as well as leadership, and following scientific development is one area in which a little of one's time can be well spent.

Risk of Decisions

Leaders set strategies (visions and goals) and tactics (objectives). You infer that good will come if people reach an end you envision and that people will reach that destination if they follow your road map. Those are big "ifs," carrying many consequences. If you are right, prosperity and health advance. If you are wrong, people suffer. Not just you and your family, but neighbors, friends, and strangers. Winston Churchill described Napoleon's march into Russia this way: "It was a brilliant strategy, marred only by failure." Napoleon lost his empire. Hundreds of thousands of his soldiers lost their lives.

Not every decision by every leader carries the same risk. A woman running a roadside fruit stand cannot be said to hold the power over people's lives of, say, a nurse in an emergency room. While the comparative game can play out in millions of ways, let us just say this: no individual aspiration compares with the desire for health. No leader, therefore, enjoys and suffers from responsibility as does the one in health care.

COMPANY BREEDS ENLIGHTENMENT

With good reason, health care systems find places on their governing boards for scientists and civic leaders. Their boards sprinkle power among experts and laity. The bank president, accountant, lawyer, and farmer sit across the table from the oncologist, radiologist, and obstetrician. No one is enslaved to the other's viewpoint. No one is more or less useful to hammering out sound policy, like buying an expensive piece of diagnostic equipment or affiliating with another health care system. As the eminent scientist and humanist Jacob Bronowski explained: "Power is the by-product of understanding."[1] The power of the health care governing board largely lies in expertise in the humanities and the sciences, forging cohesive thought and wise strategy. A health system's board of trustees probably is the best example in society where the humanities and sciences meld together, add value to the other's perspective, and forge a coherent opinion and vision.

An unsurpassed virtue of good leadership is its influence on a community's norms, standards, and behavior. Herein, trustees have a golden opportunity. They can explain to their followers, the general public, why so much medicine has shifted from inpatient to outpatient care and from invasive therapeutics to diagnostics to identifying diseases. The enlightened leadership of a health care board can help residents grapple with end-of-life and beginning-of-life trade-offs, explicit rationing of medical care, and the difference between quantity and quality of life. It takes altruism to tell residents straightforwardly that they'd be better off giving up cigarettes and doctors than keeping both.[2] It is no way to fill an acute care bed, but such advice, if taken, would certainly improve health status in the community.

EXPLORING SCIENCE

Say that you are a health care leader without a great deal of knowledge of biology and science. How much do you need to learn and how do you go about doing it? This entire book is designed to help you. What follows are some experiences I have gained and some suggestions about how you might go about the search for knowledge. (A list of further readings concludes the chapter.)

You will enjoy Howard Gardner's books on intelligence, which explore such aptitudes as sports, music, and emotional maturity—routinely foreign to course work in reading, writing, and arithmetic and certainly not revealed in testing on those subjects. Gardner proves that diverse human talents strengthen society. As we plow through the late stages of an industrial era hallmarked by standardization, it is comforting to know that humans are customized in their talents and outlooks.

Kevin Kelly's *Out of Control* is well worth reading. Kelly is the executive editor of *Wired,* an information technology magazine. Hardly alone, he foresees integration of biology and technology. He believes that humans increasingly will have machine-like properties and machines will have human-like properties. "When the union of the born and the made is complete, our fabrications will learn, adapt, heal themselves, and evolve."[3] In short, our creations will be out of our control.

How the Mind Works by Stephen Pinker, a neuroscientist at the Massachusetts Institute of Technology, surveys just how much progress has been made in understanding the physiology of the human mind. Consider the questions he answers: Why do memories fade? How does makeup change the look of a face? Where do ethnic stereotypes come from? Why do people lose their tempers? What makes children bratty? Why do fools fall in love? What makes us laugh? Why do people believe in ghosts and spirits?[4]

Biological Roots of Behavior

Hardly a day passes that an individual does not lose a memory, find someone else attractive, jump to a conclusion, get angry, become upset by someone else's behavior, think about love, laugh, or accept something that can't be proven. The work and fun of the ordinary day go on without our asking why and how. But such common, everyday behaviors have physiological roots. Nerves, neurons, synapses, the retina, and a jumble of other physical machinery produce feelings, moods, attitudes, and opinions.

Humans alone have created culture and language. That may be due to divine intervention, but we know that the capacity to create art and symbolize thoughts in language is physiologically founded. We are the only species that organizes government; arranges itself into religious, ethnic, and political camps; and devises rules to govern the tribe. Apart from social insects, only humans, chimpanzees, dolphins, and perhaps bonobos (pygmy chimpanzees) join in groups of four or more to attack others of the species—in other words, make war. These are some of the largest-brained species. Pinker bluntly reasons that "war may require sophisticated mental machinery."[5]

Humans alone create such art as paintings, plays, and music and intend to pass them on to successive generations. The human thinks about the past and future. It may be that the individual thinks more futuristically than the institutions we have organized. Certainly, politics and collective thought pay little heed to the long term. In politics as well as economics—as Bill Cooper (a Michigan State University zoologist of international repute) told me—"the future is grossly discounted." Weighing my personal best interests today against my daughter's best interests 25 years from now, I will take my daughter's side. But weighing my personal best interests today against the community's or world's best interests down the road, I take the selfish view.

If laughter, war, sexual attraction, and musical and literary appreciation have physiological roots, hospital, health care, and all other public policy hardly can be immune. If we find the brain's locus and neural network for violence (and it seems certain that we will) and embrace the medical intervention necessary to disarm them (a big if), will we need to build prisons and jails? Will we need to employ the police? Will we need government for security?

We do not have the definitive answers about the biological roots of violence. But in fields in which we do have definitive biological knowledge, human organizations are slow to act. If a four-year-old child masters foreign language much more readily than one of fifteen, why are educators waiting until middle school to introduce Spanish or French? If Viagra relieves impotency, why are many politicians and health care payers reluctant to let every man pop them as frequently as he would like? If a morning-after pill (RU 486) prevents pregnancy, why the struggle to keep the abortifacient off pharmacy shelves?

Experiences Modulate Behavior

Certainly not all behavior is genetically wired; our home, friends, television, and personal experiences modulate such predispositions as a tendency toward violence. But with regard to most human behavior—including violence—the research evidence is unrelenting: Nature (genes) carries every bit the clout of nurture (the environment). Scientists pretty much agree that about half of who I am, what I think, and how I behave is inherited through genes. The other half is shaped by other things, and here is where scientists divide.

You may have heard about the book *The Nurture Assumption*, whose author Judith Rich Harris argues that children's peers outside the home leave a greater imprint on their life than do their parents, whose dominant influence is the passing on of genes. Harris stakes out a theory she calls group socialization and makes this prediction: Children would develop into the same sort of adults if we left their lives outside the home unchanged—left them in their schools and their neighborhoods—but switched all the parents around.[6] So, get over your guilt!

Child development psychologists do not all agree with Harris. Through attachment research, many believe that the early childhood relationship between child and parents, particularly the mother, directly shapes the brain's framework. Genes provide information; early life experiences transcribe that information and affect how the genes are expressed.

Some scientists hew toward biology as the explainer of attitudes and behavior; some hew more toward the environment. Within the environment, some scientists emphasize the impact of biological or adoptive parents, while others trace behavioral roots to children's peer groups, and others to human-to-machine bonds such as television and other media.

Neuroscience is harrumphing its way toward answers. This is much the way physicists debated, negotiated, and eventually resolved differences over atomic theory. We have left the age of physics. We are in the age of biology. That does not mean that physics is irrelevant to modern life, but rather that biology is on the brink of bringing in the next 50 years the same level of consequences to health and learning that the atom and hydrogen bombs brought to world order in the past 50 years.

SCIENCE VERSUS HUMANITIES

Ideology—not scientific fact—confines society. Religion is not the only area in which rules and outcomes are fueled by belief rather than fact; this also is the essence of politics, hence the maxim that in politics all facts are negotiable. Temporizing in regard to science may not necessarily be bad. Maybe it was a bad outcome to allow Robert Oppenheimer, Enrico Fermi, and their cohort to test the atomic bomb in New Mexico in 1945, but science cannot be restrained forever. Someone would have perfected the bomb—if not the United States, another political entity.

When the Catholic Church reined in Galileo, it moved outside of its realm by seeking to have its dogma explain everything. The church could not have known that the facts that eventually would prove Galileo correct also would prove its dogma to be in error. It is not wise for a religion to fool around with temporal matters, because, as François de la Rouchefoucauld put it more than 300 years ago, "There is nothing more horrible than the murder of a beautiful theory by a gang of brutal facts." Faith works because it cannot be proven to be true or false.

I particularly appreciate the intellectual honesty of an editorial in the *Detroit News* entitled "The Cloning Panic." In commenting on the rash of legislation to ban cloning, it said:

> The potential for human cloning does raise fundamental moral questions—as have all amazing leaps in technology through history. We are, after all, dealing with the very essence of life. But overlooked in this rush to legislate is the fact that, on balance, man's manipulation of nature has vastly improved the human condition.[7]

Plodding toward truth, science does not rely on metaphysics, political interpretation, religious doctrine, or values. "The mind . . . is designed to solve many engineering problems," Pinker writes.[8] One hundred fifty years ago, Darwin was right when he concluded the *Origin of Species* with the prediction that "psychology will be based on a new foundation." Humans have frittered away most of that time in specious preoccupation with nonscientific refutations like Freudian theory and William Jennings Bryan's brand of creationism.

If you are curious about how far Darwinism has advanced in science, you might check out Richard Dawkins' *A River Out of Eden*, which boils down all life to genes and DNA. Dawkins warns that one of the hardest lessons for humans to learn is that nature is not cruel, only pitilessly indifferent. "We cannot admit that things might be neither good nor evil, neither cruel nor kind, but simply callous—indifferent to all suffering, lacking all purpose."[9] In such an unambiguous statement does science launch an all-out assault on the premise of the humanities.

Someone not schooled in medicine has difficulty understanding how a pediatric oncologist stays sane. Each day, the oncologist sees life-ending disease in children who have not had time to destroy their bodies through smoking, drinking, and overeating. Surrounded daily by premature disease and death among precious and innocent children, how can a caregiver keep going? Because the oncologist examines cell structure the way a certified public accountant examines receipts and trade payables. It makes the oncologist no less humane but fortunately for patients and families, less biased by passion.

Humans attend to both truths and beliefs, science and values. Because of the power of thought, we humans have rights that other species lack, like the right to unplug the television. Science invents; people bear consequences. As scientific advance becomes more pervasive, the consequences escalate dramatically and people must be engaged in weighing those consequences.

Science and technology are not mysteries, but surely their offspring frequently are. Even the greatest innovator of the modern age, Thomas Edison, could not envision a single use of the phonograph having to do with the playing of music. There are serendipity and mystery to human experience that are immune to all the king's horses and all the king's men. That is why we have an obligation to think through the psychological, economic, cultural, and political ramifications of innovation and to inject ethics into technology.

BIOLOGY AND HUMAN AFFAIRS

No scholar has distinguished and blurred so lucidly the boundaries of biology and ethics than Leon Kass, MD, of the University of Chicago. Reviewing the titles of his works reveals the man's tortured and inspiring attempts to reconcile science and morality: "The End of Medicine and Pursuit of Health," "Is There a Medical Ethic?" "Mortality and Morality: The Virtues of Finitude," *The New Biology: What Price Relieving Man's Estate?* "Patenting Life," "Perfect Babies: Prenatal Diagnosis and the Equal Right to Life," "Practicing Prudently: Ethical Dilemmas in Caring for the Ill," "Teleology, Darwinism, and the Place of Man: Beyond Chance and Necessity."[10]

Kass distinguishes between the pursuit of knowledge (science) and the conduct of life (ethics). The conflict has roots in intellectual conversation that is ancient (Aristotle) and persistent (Bacon, Descartes, Einstein). But as science progresses, the conflict gets so much more complicated and carries a greater stake, as Kass explains:

Science is not only methodologically indifferent to questions of better or worse. . . . The scientific findings about nature and man are not congenial to human need, self-image, or aspiration. Nature, as seen by our physicists, proceeds deterministically, without purpose or direction, utterly silent on matters of better and worse, and without a hint of guidance as to how we are to live. . . . The teachings of science, however gratifying as discoveries to the mind, throw icy waters on the human spirit.[11]

POLITICS AND SCIENCE

At the word *politics*, people shriek in horror. That damnable cesspool of corruption. Politicians, those creepy, untrustworthy rascals. Imitate Howard Deale, who vented in the movie *Network:* "Get up now, out of your chairs, get up right now and go to the window. Open it. Stick your head out. Yell, I'm mad as hell, and I'm not going to take this anymore."[12] Go ahead. Get your hatred of politics out of your system. Then, let's think about the importance of politics.

Politics is governance. Be it national, state, local, neighborhood, civic board, or health care system's board of trustees, politics balances points of view and goes a lot further. It morphs those views, usually widely disparate, into a coherent set of values. It goes further still. It enforces those values on every member of the tribe. When the greater number of the tribe decides to change values, politics is the device by which we peacefully alter course.

Politics is what leaders practice. You practice it in your board or committee meeting. Without politics, you would not make policy as a group. You simply would awake each morning and all on your own decide how to spend money and foist your rules on everyone else.

Politics is the fulcrum of a teeter-totter. On one seat there's a 200-pound guy screaming that abortion is wrong. Opposite is a 110-pound gal screaming that she has every right to abort. But it is not just "mano-a-womano." This teeter-totter has 100,000 seats in your community, one for every resident. Everybody weighs the same. The fulcrum—politics—does not follow a principle that one seat must be in the air and the other on the ground. It seeks equilibrium. Every teeter-totter sitter is about the same level off the ground.

Politics is the natural fulcrum to bring equilibrium between science and religion, each of which abhors negotiation. Science explores only fact. Religion harbors no fact. Science explains how humans and nature work. When science lacks an answer, religion fills it. Politics balances fact and opinion and then goes on to balance all differing opinions. Sometimes to balance opinions, it tosses out facts. It tosses out anything that may cause one teeter-totter seat to lurch into the air. It drives endlessly toward equilibrium. Its end result, which is public policy, may not always seem coherent or rational, moral or unjust. It seeks to minimize how incoherent, irrational, immoral, and unjust any one group feels toward the resolution.

As schoolchildren in America, we learn that our society stands for life, liberty, and the pursuit of happiness. How has scientific invention advanced these human goals? Penicillin extends life. The morning-after pill snuffs it out. Airplanes free us from travel exclusively on ground or sea. The beeper and cell phone restrain our enjoyment of leisure. Antidepressants allow us to see the world as less dark and frightening. The threat of atomic warfare taught 1950s' children that happiness stopped at the fallout shelter. Politics mediates science, just as the environment mediates the propensity of genes. Through group discussion, the effects of science are considered. Neurons and ethics cohabit this space.

Health is the doctor's business. Life, liberty, and the pursuit of happiness are the business of everyone. Health is a scientific state of being. Life, liberty, and the pursuit of happiness are human and political rights. Medicine does not determine health. Self-governance determines life, liberty, and the pursuit of happiness. What separates humans from other creatures is the loftiness and breadth of our thinking and goals. The frog is programmed to maintain its species within the bounds that nature provides. Humans are programmed to maintain their species and free to frame and alter behavior before, during, and after propagation. Nature is all-determining to the frog. Nature is partly determining to human beings.

AGE OF ENLIGHTENMENT

A lofty ideal is to have the humanities and science live at peace with one another. There was a time when they were not at war: when politics was driven by science, and ideology and fact coexisted. That time is called the Age of Enlightenment, which spanned the seventeenth and eighteenth centuries. Rousseau's philosophy, Descartes's mathematics principles, Marat's revolutionary fervor, America's founders' pursuit of liberty, Galileo's and Newton's physics findings, and Watt's steam engine all converged in Western civilization. Men saw political freedom as a natural outgrowth of scientific knowledge. Morality was grounded in reason.

To survive this era, religions (for the most part) wisely declined to fight science's integration into culture. Monarchs, however, took another view—Louis XVI of France and George III of England unwisely decided to battle it out with their malcontents. The religious institutions lived on, but the kingdoms crumbled. Democracy was created in part by ideology and faith; it was also created by an industrial economy fed by scientific findings that made tyranny only ephemerally effective in restraining individual freedom. The political drive was indeed as pitilessly indifferent as Dawkins describes nature to be.

We purport to be smarter than those who preceded us, but what has it gotten us? During the past century we have permitted—or driven—any number of disciplines (physics is a good example) to isolate themselves artificially from the mainstream; we confine them primarily to academia, where the practitioners speak to each other in a language only they can understand, in part because the rest of us do not listen to what they have to say. We have permitted philosopher-kings, such as Marx and Freud, to rule the arts and even many of the sciences. We have permitted the evolution of the most tyrannical states seen in world history and witnessed more vile human warfare than has occurred in any other time. We drain Earth of scarce natural resources. We selfishly discharge effluent into our waters, spill poison onto our lands, and excrete toxicities into our fragile atmosphere. We educate children in a way not much different from that of a hundred years ago, ignoring what we have learned about the physiology of the human brain.

Politics is about the search for comfort in the present, as alluded to earlier. Which candidate—what policy—will make us safer and better educated today without spending any more of our hard-earned dollars? It certainly is not criminal to think of oneself and take stock of how life is treating us today, but leaders—and not just political ones—have a loftier responsibility: to impart to their corner of society a sense of direction that will carry us into the future and require us to change.

In leadership, ignorance never is bliss. To know that the human body is programmed to (1) maximize its chances of living until it is old enough to propagate the species and (2) decline after the age of reproduction, becoming subject to myriad life-ending chronic diseases, is to challenge the notion that all medicine, at all ages, is a right. Desirable, humane, compassionate—yes. But a physiological right? No. Science can tell us that once past our capacity to reproduce—that is, after we have assured that the species and our personal DNA will be carried on—we are not naturally entitled to medical care; politics certainly cannot. But what if leaders of science, politics, religion, and medicine were to come together and blend science and belief, and the lust for present gratification and Earth's future accommodation of a finite number of people? (Consider, for example, the environmental writer Bill McKibben's calculation that if Americans died in this century at the same rate as they did in 1900, the population of our country would stand at 140 million, not 270 million.)

The Brink Of Enlightenment

One of the world's preeminent biologists and writers, Edward O. Wilson, has produced a work of rare optimism and brilliance entitled *Consilience*. This eighteenth-century word suggests a coming together—a bridging—of science and the humanities. A summary cannot do justice to the profundity and hope of Wilson's book. The book calls us to action.

It is as pointless and counterproductive to take ideology out of politics as it is to take facts out of science. Nonetheless, there is a benefit to politics using, weighing, and explaining to the public more scientific fact—and, in turn, science using and considering philosophy, morality, and the human factor. Any institution benefits from taking into account science's longer view; science benefits from taking into account the difficulty in trading short-term gain for long-term improvement.

Scientists—who can be as haughty and off-putting as any ideologue—should come out of their labs and converse with the public. The public's leaders need to welcome them and help them to translate their findings for the general audience. Science can be a masterful instrument in causing people to assume a perspective about human health and well-being that extends beyond their family unit. Scientists must be mindful, however, of the fallout from their "good" news: When, as occurs from time to time, a newspaper headline proclaims that a cure for cancer is only two years away, the hundreds of thousands of cancer patients with 18 months to live can only feel devastated by the fates.

Enlightenment in Your Community

Enlightenment presumes that leaders, followers, and scientists listen to one another and weigh matters. In most communities, such conversation never occurs. One reason is that people do not think to do it. Another hurdle is that people do not think that they control the march of science.

Health care leaders simply acquiesce to the community's medical fate being determined by innovation, policies, and regulation foisted on it from elsewhere. Most communities do not house eminent research scientists and medical research. Medical marvels seep into town after trials and tests in a Geneva laboratory. Whether or not—and how much—the health care system gets reimbursed for using technology in diagnosis and therapy is controlled by state governments and the federal government or big insurance companies headquartered miles away. The community does not limit or extend access to medications; that's the job of the Food and Drug Administration.

Enter devolution. End excuses. Bring on community involvement and enlightenment. America is moving rapidly toward devolution of power: from Washington, DC, to state capitols, and from there to counties, cities, villages, and townships, and from these to neighborhoods and homes. Concentrated power increasingly smells a lot like factory effluence, a relic of an industrial age. One hallmark after another of the industrial age is falling and being replaced by new paradigms. Efficiency is losing out to personal freedom. Standardization is losing out to customization. Hierarchies are being dismantled into small hubs.

Power isn't all that it's cracked up to be. Health care leaders will shoulder more responsibility than ever before. They must start acting purposefully rather than reacting to outside events. Followers will have to be smarter consumers and shrewder customers. Scientists, most notably the medical profession, must be educators and draw their communities into discussion of explicit ethical choices.

I offer a variety of suggestions that could make your community one that is truly enlightened.

WHAT CAN HEALTH CARE LEADERS DO?

1. Place on the agenda of every meeting a discussion of science and ethics. Alternate between clinicians and nonclinicians as

topic leaders. Do not be afraid of discussing tough issues, but make sure that everyone's opinion and knowledge of fact are welcome and heard. The discussion does not always have to be a debate over how much your health care system spends on little children as opposed to seniors or abortion policy. More often than not, this discussion will take the form of a presentation by a physician, nurse, or other clinician that brings the group up to speed on new research endeavors and findings.

2. Ensure that there is a director of education or chief information officer responsible for helping you and other leaders learn about medical science. Some of us have participated in book clubs where members gather and discuss reflections on the same book. That is what I have in mind. If every month, a board, having been assigned an article or book, came together for an hour or two and shared company and perspectives, the effect on policymaking would be extraordinary.

3. Require community impact statements before technology is purchased and put to use. Consider the factors of how evenly distributed access to the technology will be; how it will affect cost of care; how it will affect patients' expectations of longevity and overall health; and who will inform the public about its benefits, drawbacks, and consequences.

4. Publish, broadcast, cablecast, and retail information about medical advances. Through all means available, help the public (1) understand scientific achievements and innovations; (2) draw reasonable expectations about their effect on personal health; and (3) engage in weighing ethical, cultural, political, and psychological consequences.

5. Evaluate Internet sources of health care information and steer consumers toward Web sites that are reliable. Appreciate that information technology, most notably the Internet and cable television, is arming your neighbors with more information than most physicians had at their fingertips 20 years ago. In the knowledge race, the gap between consumers and experts in medicine is declining by the week. Smarter consumers will be smarter buyers of health care. They also will be critical thinkers, questioning authority, demanding second and third opinions. Many will come to the physician's office or hospital

armed with tabloid-quality misinformation about technologies, marvels, medications, and cures. Health care leaders must help their community's members separate the wheat from the chaff.

6. Sponsor presentations on medical science before civic groups. By extending knowledge to residents and other leaders in your community, you will be arming them to become smarter consumers. You will be amazed at their level of interest, intelligent questions, and eagerness for take-home information.

7. Sponsor a medicine and community ethics panel. Assemble leaders of religious faiths, physicians, heads of charitable groups, educators, and political leaders to meet a couple of times each year to share opinions and facts about medical miracles and their impact on the community's faiths, economy, culture, and psychology. Your community newspaper will be a helpful partner, providing coverage to the deliberations and providing readers with an exchange of knowledge and opinions.

CONCLUSION

I, unlike some, happen to think that people are on the brink of a new age of enlightenment, in which science and the arts will join forces. I look forward to leaders heeding science and science heeding public opinion. Humans will embrace machines and resemble them. Machines will exhibit such human-like qualities as logic. Most important, people will rally around a code of behavior and values that accept scientific principles and facts, and scientific investigation will teach us how to preserve nature and prolong its capacity to nourish *Homo sapiens*.

The world need not be myopic, brutal, and vulgar. Nurture and nature need not contest over the mastery of life. Our health care, civic, business, and political leaders need not be laughed out of service because they consider science; scientists need not be shut away in academia like the proverbial crazy relative hidden in the attic.

The wearisome caveats about things outside our community's control are giving way to a new philosophy grounded in "why not" and "what works for us." It is time for conversation. It is time for consilience. The right place for consilience is within our communities.

References

1. Jacob Bronowski, *Science and Human Values* (New York: Harper & Row, 1992), p. 10.

2. Thomas McKeown, *The Role of Medicine* (Princeton, NJ: Princeton University Press, 1980).

3. Kevin Kelley, *Out of Control* (Reading, MA: Addison-Wesley, 1994).

4. Stephen Pinker, *How the Mind Works* (New York: W. W. Norton, 1997), p. 3.

5. Ibid., p. 513.

6. Judith Rich Harris, *The Nurture Assumption: Why Children Turn Out the Way They Do* (New York: Free Press, 1998), p. 359.

7. "The Cloning Panic," *Detroit News* (February 8, 1998): B6.

8. Pinker, *How the Mind Works*, p. 4.

9. Richard Dawkins, *A River Out of Eden* (New York: Basic Books, 1995), p. 96.

10. "Credits" in Leon Kass, *Toward a More Natural Science: Biology and Human Affairs* (New York: Basic Books, 1995), p. v.

11. Kass, *Toward a More Natural Science*, pp. 5–6.

12. *Network*, Sidney Lumet, MGM, 1976.

Bibliography

Brockman, John. *The Third Culture: Beyond the Scientific Revolution* (New York: Simon & Schuster, 1996).

Denning, Peter J., and Robert M. Metcalfe. *Beyond Calculation: The Next Fifty Years of Computing* (New York: Springer-Verlag, 1997).

Gardner, Howard. *Art, Mind, and Brain: A Cognitive Approach to Creativity* (New York: Basic Books, 1982).

————. *Frames of Mind: The Theories of Multiple Intelligences* (New York: Basic Books, 1993).

————. *Multiple Intelligences: The Theory in Practice* (New York: Basic Books, 1993).

Goleman, Daniel. *Emotional Intelligence* (New York: Bantam Books, 1997).

Kaku, Michio. *Visions: How Science Will Revolutionize the 21st Century* (New York: Anchor Books, 1997).

Rothschild, Michael. *Bionomics: Economy as Ecosystem* (New York: Henry Holt, 1990).

Sclove, Richard E. *Democracy and Technology* (New York: Guilford Press, 1995).

Tapscott, Don. *The Digital Economy: Promise and Peril in the Age of Networked Intelligence* (New York: McGraw-Hill, 1996).

Wilson, Edward O. *Consilience* (New York: Alfred A. Knopf, 1998).

CHAPTER 13

EPILOGUE: A POSTSCRIPT ON PROGRESS

P rogress is progress, right? It's what happens when things advance, get better.

Not at all. It's a "noxious, culturally embedded, untestable, nonoperational, intractable idea that must be replaced if we wish to understand the patterns of history," according to Stephen Jay Gould.[1] Whew!

Fortunately for our sanity, Dr. Gould is expressing no more than his opinion, and it can mercifully be ignored. Julian Huxley (1887–1975), brother of *Brave New World* author Aldous and architect of the modern synthesis of Darwinian natural selection with Mendelian genetics, had a more attractive opinion:

> The scientific doctrine of progress . . . will inevitably become one of the cornerstones of man's theology, or whatever may be the future substitute for theology, and the most important external support for human ethics.[2]

A biologist, like Gould, Huxley focused on progress in the biological world—in evolution, to be more precise. He believed that progress was inevitable but unpredictable. In evolution, species that developed better sensory and manipulative organs would have either greater control over their environment or greater independence of it.

Humankind became dominant in both respects but only partially for bioevolutionary reasons. The eagle has sharper eyes than we do, the bat sharper ears, the ape more strength, the cheetah more speed, the dog a keener sense of smell. Our advantage lay, first, in being generalists rather than specialists, and, second, in our unique development of language, which enabled general knowledge to be shared and stored—to accumulate—over successive generations.

All of this is just another way of saying that memetics—the evolution of ideas—is an advance on, or progress over, genetics. But suppose you took all the advantages of both the specialist and the generalist—the ability to spot a mouse whisker from a thousand feet in the air, to smell a sparrow's fart in a pig sty, to hear the flap of a butterfly wing on 5th Avenue in rush hour, to see inside objects with x-ray vision, to smell their chemical composition; and the ability then to accumulate and generalize from the resultant sensory data and experiences, collating them with previously accumulated knowledge to arrive at more refined interpretations and—and you have Superwo/man, or *Machina sapiens*, or a symbiont of both: a cyborg. For certain, you have progress.

Still not convinced? How about the speed with which biological neural nets respond to stimuli? Over the course of evolution, Huxley informs us, "the speed at which messages are transmitted along nerve fibers has increased over six hundredfold, from below six inches a second in some nerve nets to over a hundred yards a second in parts of our own nervous system." Which sounds like impressive progress—until you consider that *Machina sapiens'* neural net operates at close to 186,000 miles a second.

As J. B. S. Haldane wrote: "Man of today is probably an extremely primitive and imperfect type of rational being."[3]

Haldane also recognized the inevitability of the reintroduction of values into supposedly value-free science, which I think is the crux of the problem some scientists, such as Gould and George Gaylord Simpson (1902–1984), have with the notion of progress.

"When we speak of progress in Evolution," wrote Haldane, "we are already leaving the relatively firm ground of scientific objectivity for the shifting morass of human values." Julian Huxley asserted that "[h]uman values are doubtless essential criteria for the steps of any future progress," and they become operative when we formulate goals. Then: "Human purpose and the progress based upon it must also take account of human needs and limitations, whether these be of a biological order, such as our dietary requirements or our mode of reproduction, or of a human order, such as our intellectual limitations or our inevitable subjection to emotional conflict." We must resolve the conflict between spiritualism and materialism, because we have been entrusted with, and must plan for, the future unfolding of evolution, and unless our inner conflict is resolved, there can be no consistent plan.

Concisely summing the key messages of Jesuit ecologist Pierre Teilhard de Chardin's universal consciousness,[4] physicist Frank Tipler's cosmic development,[5] and biologist Richard Dawkins' memetics,[6] Huxley added:

> In the light of evolutionary biology man can now see himself as the sole agent of further evolutionary advance on this planet, and one of the few possible instruments of progress in the universe at large. He finds himself in the unexpected position of business manager for the cosmic process of evolution. He no longer ought to feel separated from the rest of nature, for he is part of it—that part which has become conscious, capable of love and understanding and aspiration. He need no longer regard himself as insignificant in relation to the cosmos. He is intensely significant. In his person, he has acquired meaning, for he is constantly creating new meanings. Human society generates new mental and spiritual agencies, and sets them to work in the cosmic process: it controls matter by means of mind.
>
> Biology has thus revealed man's place in nature. He is the highest form of life produced by the evolutionary process on this planet, the latest dominant type, and the only organism capable of further major advance or progress. His destiny is to realize new possibilities for the whole terrestrial sector of the cosmic process, to be the instrument of further evolutionary progress on this planet.[7]

The developments described in this book show that Huxley was more right than probably even he imagined.

References

1. Quoted in Connie Barlow, ed., *Evolution Extended: Biological Debates on the Meaning of Life* (Cambridge, MA: The MIT Press, 1994), p. 50. For a recent example of Gould's antiprogress theorizing, see Stephen J. Gould, *Full House: The Spread of Excellence from Plato to Darwin* (New York: Three Rivers Press, 1996).

2. Julian Huxley, *New Bottles for New Wine* (London: Harper & Row, 1957), p. 21.

3. Quoted in Barlow, *Evolution Extended*, p. 17.

4. Pierre Teilhard de Chardin, *The Phenomenon of Man* (New York: Harper Brothers, 1959).

5. Frank J. Tipler, *The Physics of Immortality: Modern Cosmology, God and the Resurrection of the Dead* (New York: Doubleday, 1994).

6. Described in Richard Dawkins, *The Blind Watchmaker: Why the Evidence of Evolution Reveals a Universe without Design* (New York: W. W. Norton, 1987).

7. Barlow, *Evolution Extended*, pp. 19–20.

Printed and bound by CPI Group (UK) Ltd, Croydon, CR0 4YY

27/10/2024

14580315-0002